Mental Health in Historical Perspective

Series Editors
Catharine Coleborne
School of Humanities and Social Science
University of Newcastle
Callaghan, NSW, Australia

Matthew Smith
Centre for the Social History of Health and Healthcare
University of Strathclyde
Glasgow, UK

Covering all historical periods and geographical contexts, the series explores how mental illness has been understood, experienced, diagnosed, treated and contested. It will publish works that engage actively with contemporary debates related to mental health and, as such, will be of interest not only to historians, but also mental health professionals, patients and policy makers. With its focus on mental health, rather than just psychiatry, the series will endeavour to provide more patient-centred histories. Although this has long been an aim of health historians, it has not been realised, and this series aims to change that.

The scope of the series is kept as broad as possible to attract good quality proposals about all aspects of the history of mental health from all periods. The series emphasises interdisciplinary approaches to the field of study, and encourages short titles, longer works, collections, and titles which stretch the boundaries of academic publishing in new ways.

More information about this series at
http://www.palgrave.com/gp/series/14806

Catharine Coleborne

Why Talk About Madness?

Bringing History into the Conversation

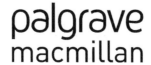

Catharine Coleborne
School of Humanities and Social
Science
University of Newcastle
Callaghan, NSW, Australia

Mental Health in Historical Perspective
ISBN 978-3-030-21095-3   ISBN 978-3-030-21096-0   (eBook)
https://doi.org/10.1007/978-3-030-21096-0

Cover credit: ian nolan/Alamy Stock Photo

This Palgrave Macmillan imprint is published by the registered company Springer Nature
Switzerland AG
The registered company address is: Gewerbestrasse 11, 6330 Cham, Switzerland

PREFACE

For more than twenty years, I have been writing about aspects of the history of madness and institutions. My scholarship has had a focus on the nineteenth-century hospitals in Australia and New Zealand which were shaped by the processes of colonialism. My work has raised questions about how institutions reflected colonial society's anxieties and preoccupations and also how societies in formation in turn produced institutional populations. In particular, my research has sought to address the interactions of patients, families and the cultures of institutions. Over time I have also increasingly been drawn into more contemporary projects about mental health which present new and different challenges. These themes and challenges are the subjects of this book. Over the past decade or more, historians and cultural theorists have examined the problem of madness, stimulated by the pace and scope of deinstitutionalisation, mental health advocacy, failures of policy and practice, the action research mode of disability studies and the rise of the mad movement. There are many vibrant and innovative past and present international research symposia, conferences and workshops on madness, as this book describes. Mental health consumer advocates have identified new themes for research and commentary, among them the institutional and treatment responses to madness and mental breakdown; the role of power in groups; the differences between compulsory or recovery treatment approaches; stigma, discrimination and social exclusion; and the impact of the mad movement itself. My hope is that this short book stimulates some new thinking about the relationships between histories of madness and its institutions, and talking about madness in public and private life.

Callaghan, Australia   Catharine Coleborne

ACKNOWLEDGEMENTS

This book emerges from a long period of time spent researching the histories of mental health and institutions in colonial Australia and New Zealand. It was during my academic work in New Zealand that my ideas about the present context for writing the histories of mental illness began to shape new research questions and directions. I am grateful to the team of mental health professionals, graduate students, and colleagues who helped me grow new ideas in that context, including members of the Tokanui project team. A workshop focused on talking about mental health in the present, held at the University of Waikato in 2014, also created space for a meaningful dialogue about scholarly directions with colleagues including Barbara Brookes, Bronwyn Labrum, Mary O'Hagan, Jim Marbrook and Kate Prebble. That workshop was funded by the University of Waikato's Faculty of Arts and Social Sciences strategic pilot research fund.

I thank especially mental health advocate Mary O'Hagan, who generously offered her time to me. In particular, I acknowledge Mary O'Hagan's permission to use excerpts of my interview with her in May of 2015 in this book. An abbreviated interview text was published as Mary O'Hagan, 'Madness in New Zealand' in *Asylum: The Magazine for Democratic Psychiatry* (2017).

My 'New Professor Talk' at the University of Newcastle in Australia in July 2016 allowed me to focus these concepts under the title 'Why Talk About Madness?', giving me the impetus for this book. I appreciate the research assistance provided by Dr. Jan McLeod, and thank my colleagues at the University of Newcastle in the School of Humanities and Social Science for their responses to this work, including Dr. Elizabeth Roberts-Pedersen and Dr. Robyn Dunlop. I have also been creatively and very ably supported by Maria Gardiner at iThinkwell.

My international colleagues in histories of mental illness, health and institutions have been profoundly important to my intellectual development. Colleagues in Canada and the UK have always been ready to offer critical and stimulating feedback during research and conference visits. Some of the material in this book was rehearsed in invited seminar presentations and papers, including those delivered at McMaster University, Ontario (Canada) in 2013; at the Society of the Social History of Medicine conference 'Disease, Health and the State', held in Oxford (England) in 2014; and at the Centre for the Social History of Health and Healthcare, University of Strathclyde in Glasgow (Scotland) in 2015.

My own forays into the scholarship of 'mad' histories are necessarily limited due to my in-between status as an academic historian, rather than an insider. I thank Geoffrey Reaume and Megan Davies, both of whom were quietly encouraging of my ability to bridge this divide during my visit to Canada in 2013. I acknowledge Dr. Rob Ellis and colleagues who organised the important 'Voices of Madness' conference, held at Huddersfield in September 2016, as well as speakers at that conference. My keynote address at that conference, 'Talk, Dissent, Silence: Narrating Madness in the Twentieth Century', forms the basis of some of this book. I also thank the four peer reviewers of the proposal for this book and the two manuscript readers for their thoughtful and incisive critiques which helped me to sharpen the focus of this provocation.

This book signals the projected outcomes of an Australian Research Council Discovery Project (DP190103655) with colleagues at the University of Sydney (2019–2021): 'The development of Australian community psychiatry'.

ABOUT THIS BOOK

The history of madness remains one of the most vibrant and controversial fields in the social history of medicine. This short book explains why we should talk more about madness in our present, but also in historical context. Using histories of madness, the book also argues that we need to imagine new ways of thinking about madness. This book is not a general text. Instead, it aims to be a provocation. *Why Talk About Madness?* argues that the story of the social and cultural impact of the history of the mad movement, self-help and mental health consumer advocacy from the 1960s must be read inside a longer tradition of first-person accounts of madness. The people at the centre of the historical narrative of mental health—those with lived experiences of madness, especially those who have been in institutional 'care' and treatment regimes—should be the focus of its histories. Starting with a brief history of the relevance of first-person accounts, and then turning to the significance of other ways of representing the 'patient', 'inmate' or 'consumer' over time, this book argues that the confinement of madness in the asylum produced specific evidence and understandings about mental health that have persisted long after the closure of asylums. It challenges this mode of understanding and presents new thinking about mental illness experiences in historical perspective that could reshape our interpretation of mental health in the present.

CONTENTS

1 Why Talk About Madness?   1

2 Asylum Archives and Cases as Stories   15

3 The Asylum and Its Afterlife   29

4 Extra-Institutional Care, or Madness Uncontained   41

5 Talking About Mental Health and the Politics of Madness   53

6 What's the Story?   65

Appendix A: Mad Studies Conferences, Symposia
            and Events, 2014–2019   73

Appendix B: Mad Studies Networks and Social Media   75

Index   79

About the Author

Catharine Coleborne is a professor, historian and is currently the Head of School of Humanities and Social Science at the University of Newcastle, New South Wales, Australia. Her books include *Madness in the Family* (Palgrave, 2010), and *Insanity, Identity and Empire* (Manchester University Press, 2015). Catharine is currently second Chief Investigator on two Australian Research Council Discovery Projects focused on histories of mental health and psychiatry in Australia spanning the nineteenth and twentieth centuries. Her next book, *Narrating Madness in the Twentieth Century*, focuses on the overarching histories of consumer networks, advocacy, policy changes, shared histories and points of difference across Australia, New Zealand, the United Kingdom and Canada. With Elizabeth Roberts-Pedersen, she is also writing a book about the global history of mental health: *Making Mental Health: A Global History* (Routledge Critical Approaches to Health).

CHAPTER 1

Why Talk About Madness?

This book provokes new conversations about madness and its histories. In his 1987 book *A Social History of Madness: The World Through the Eyes of the Insane*, historian Roy Porter presented a powerful critique of psychiatry: he suggested that psychiatrists had effectively 'excommunicated the mad from human society, even when their own cries and complaints have been human' (Porter 1987, 233). Since Porter wrote, historians, governments, communities, psychiatric experts and the mad themselves have continued to ask questions about institutional care, psychiatric treatments and diagnoses, and about what it means to be mad. In the present, what we need is more dialogue: to listen, hear and engage across the borders of madness and its care, or what Porter termed 'madness and psychiatry talking' (Porter 1987, 8).

In this way, then, this book is part of a much longer public and scholarly discussion about madness. It takes selected evidence from different places across the international landscape of mental health following post-war institutional closures, but concentrates mostly on what we might term the British world, a site which has a shared history of mental health approaches, policy and practice. It presents short case studies from Britain, Australia, New Zealand and Canada to illustrate larger points about the impact of deinstitutionalisation on our thinking about madness in history (Kritsotaki et al. 2016, 6–7; 23). In doing so, this book signals the need for a more detailed transnational global story of mental illness, one that aims to connect the various interventions made into mental health care over time by mental health advocates, those with lived

© The Author(s) 2020
C. Coleborne, *Why Talk About Madness?* Mental Health in Historical Perspective, https://doi.org/10.1007/978-3-030-21096-0_1

experience of madness, and professional experts interested in the mad themselves.

Continuing the provocation by Porter, and fashioned as a response to the growing international field of 'mad studies', this book provides a historical interpretation of the critique of the history of psychiatry over time. Mad studies are credited in recent times with bringing a 'voice of sanity' to the field of psychiatry (Beresford 2014). Scholars interested in the field of mad studies have set out a new activist framework for the writing of histories of madness (see *Mad Matters*, LeFrançois, Menzies and Reaume, eds 2013). *Mad Matters* examines the field of mad studies from a range of disciplinary perspectives. It uses the idea of 'mad people's history'—a history prompted by the mad movement and legacies of anti-psychiatry—and it takes the theme of narratives, telling stories about sanity and madness. It also mounts a series of critiques of psychiatry, engaging with law, public policy and media, as well as with questions of social justice and identity politics. The editors assert that the field of mad studies offers both a new critical framework and an exercise in critical pedagogy, also circulating new knowledge and ideas about mental illness to contest regimes of 'truth' (LeFrançois, Menzies and Reaume, eds 2013, 14).

Although this idea is faintly echoed in Andrew Scull's weighty volume about madness, *Madness in Civilisation* (2015), Scull does not go far enough with his analysis of why, or how, madness needs to be rearticulated (see Coleborne 2017, 428). Porter was clearer about his efforts to retrieve the patients' voices in histories of medicine, and had offered several examples of the voices of the 'mad' in his many works of history. Porter suggested that he was keen to discover 'what mad people meant to say, what was on their minds' (Porter 1987, 1). In a deftly argued chapter of his *Brief History* (2002), he suggested that influential histories of psychiatry had encouraged scholars to stop listening to the mad (157). The striving for some form of 'objective' view of mental illness within the medical model led to a sharp breaking off from those asylum studies that were seeking to understand the circumstances of committal and the worlds of patients. All of this is supported by newer grassroots movements to engage survivors, mental health service consumers and users, and those with lived experiences such as the 'Hearing Voices' network in the UK, emerging from the 1980s, as well as World Health Organization (WHO) global mental health priorities in recent years.

One motivation for all of this work lies in redressing the problem of the profound silencing of the stories of mental illness by those who have experienced it, and the controlling effect of the powerful, monolithic institution of psychiatry and its asylums and hospitals that spanned the nineteenth and twentieth centuries. In her piece about silences and psychiatry, historian Diana Gittins writes that 'Not just social groups, but also historical eras can become cloaked in silence' (1998b, 47). Silences shaped our understanding of institutions, their inhabitants, and their histories, until these were opened up to scrutiny, a process that was hastened by institutional closures. Gittins was writing about Severalls Hospital in Essex at the time of its closure in 1997, a closure running parallel to that of a New Zealand institution I have also examined, Tokanui Hospital in the Waikato region of the North Island. Both places were immersed in the worlds of their wider communities; they were significant in the lives of large numbers of people for almost the whole of the twentieth century. Their shared past also points to the profound influence of British psychiatry and its institutions on the former colonies, and the impact of imperial world concepts of medical and psychiatric treatment on British world populations, including the colonised.

As this book explains, New Zealand provides a useful point of difference in its approach to mental health policy, institutional closures, consumer advocacy and more, as well as its focus on positive Māori mental health in recent years. The concept of 'Whai Ora', or a 'meshing [of] Māori values with Western medical treatment', developed over time from a 'cultural therapy unit' at Tokanui Hospital in New Zealand's North Island (Diamond 2005, 32; Durie 1994). Like New Zealand, both Australia and Canada suggest different nodes of the British world of mental health, inflected by common histories of colonisation, Indigenous peoples' experiences of psychiatric institutions and influences from both the Commonwealth and the Anglo-American world of psychiatric treatment. One original aspect of this book lies in its insistence on the value of considering perspectives from the histories of colonialism and madness, a theme that is highlighted in each chapter.

It is my view that the asylum was a *social institution* which created definitions and reflections of madness in place and space (Coleborne 2015, 7). In the 1960s, the French philosopher Michel Foucault argued that it was the institution of the asylum which brought insanity into view. He went as far as suggesting that 'Perhaps some day we will no longer really know what madness was. Its face will have closed upon itself, no longer allowing us to decipher the traces it may have left behind' (Foucault, trans. 1995, 290). The asylum was therefore much more than a building. It was a whole world, one with a hierarchy of staff, separate wards, corridors, farms and gardens, a system, where power was held by doctors and attendants. As Gittins (1998a) has noted, the 'home and harbour' meaning of the asylum (27–28), was a space conceived at a particular time (3), for specific purposes and practices. Oliver Sacks' elegant essay 'The Lost Virtues of the Asylum' captures the ambivalent identity of an institution whose meanings changed over time: 'we forgot the benign aspects of asylums, or perhaps we felt we could no longer afford to pay for them' (Sacks 2019 [2009], 192).

This institutional system also created official records required by law and imagined through medical practice. Records were administrative traces of knowledge about individuals who were confined for later generations of us to discover and puzzle over. These 'black marks' of the institutional case notes of mental illness, as Foucault mused, might be its only evidence over time—the fact that it was written about, that the utterances and physical behaviours of the mad were recorded. The mad themselves had less power to write or recount their experiences, although many accounts are extant. On balance, it is apparent that the institution has held a deeply pronounced power to *represent* madness over time, as evidenced by the critique of the medical model of mental illness in the work of Thomas Szasz in *The Myth of Mental Illness* (Szasz 1961). This view was also espoused by the anti-psychiatry movement of 1964–1970s (Crossley 1998, 886). Later incarnations of anti-psychiatry have remained true to the call by prominent psychoanalyst and anti-psychiatry figure, R. D. Laing, to understand the nature of madness (Crossley and Crossley 2001, 1487).

Such institutional power has made the present task to find, disentangle and represent histories of patient experience, as well as stories of abuses and of institutional violence, very difficult. This goes for psychiatric survivors, mental health consumers, mental health service-users, and those with lived experience, as much as it goes for the historian or sociologist, or any researcher trying to reveal, expose or share such histories for public consumption. These terms are historically specific, part of a larger 'mental health movement' emerging in the twentieth century (Crossley and Crossley 2001, 1487). Such language is important, and speaks to the way that powerful identities have been forged through shared experience and a 'process of struggle' in the formation of a lived

identity or habitus (Crossley and Crossley 2001, 1487). 'Psychiatric survivors' is a descriptor given to people who railed against the locked institutions of the 1960s and 1970s, but who emerged as having survived
the sometimes violent total institution; 'survivor' is a powerful term in
the context of post-war recognition of the horrors of the Holocaust. The
term retains its significance through current manifestations of movements such as #MeToo. Mental health 'consumers' is a term made popular in the 1980s as health systems oriented around consumer needs and
behaviours, a trend which also prompted new histories of 'the patient'
in the period. Mental health 'service-users' speaks to the idea that 'consumer' is a loaded category; many people have used or accessed services
without constituting themselves as having the freedom or agency of a
private consumer. Most recently, 'lived experience' denotes the broader
sense of madness in our communities as experienced by those who may
not have been hospitalised but who experience mental illness, and who
may or may not access services or forms of treatment. These terms are
used in this book in ways which speak to their specific historical contexts
and meanings in place.

The practical and intellectual work to fully comprehend what it
means to be mad is ongoing, and the political advocacy of and for the
mad themselves now plays a central role in that work, as several chapters in this book explain. In addition, as scholars in the field also note,
reclaiming the term 'madness' for this volume allows me to examine its
meanings in the present, as well as gesture towards a continuity of experiences of the mad and institutionalised from the past. The book shows
that those people experiencing mental illness, including some who were
the former inhabitants of the large psychiatric institutions described in
the proliferation of academic and institutional histories from the 1960s
onwards, tell somewhat different stories from those who have often
shaped official and academic histories of mental health, and it historicises
these narratives.

The central argument of this book is that the stories from those with
lived experience are vital to contemporary histories of mental health.
Without such views or voices, histories of psychiatry and its treatments
lose power and intelligibility. It was at the critical juncture of institutional
closures in the final quarter of the twentieth century that the possibility
for new thinking about histories of mental health and institutions col-
lided with social histories of the vast archive of the nineteenth-century
asylum. That is to say, the availability of new ways of seeing inside older

histories of the monolithic institution has come to challenge, in profound ways, accepted truths about the history of psychiatry. Here, I aim to address the inherent problem of historians and others continuing to perpetuate the negative and troubling representations or stereotypes of mental illness, and the possibilities for *alternative* representations as we continue to uncover historical evidence. Because madness has been 'contained' in writing about institutions, the next phase of its articulation lies in new ways to examine the past of mental breakdown beyond the confines of institutional walls.

The book also draws on an oral interview I conducted with an international consultant in mental health recovery and wellbeing, New Zealand-based Mary O'Hagan, who was the first chairperson of the World Network of Users and Survivors of Psychiatry in the 1990s. A peer advocate and award-winning author (*Madness Made Me: A Memoir*, 2014), O'Hagan worked as an advisor to the United Nations and World Health Organization and served as one of three Mental Health Commissioners in New Zealand between 2000 and 2007. Mary discussed the view that 'madness' has been seen as a stigmatising word; she argued that it is 'a reclaimed word', and also a 'lay word ... a common everyday word ... a replacement word for what people call serious mental illness' (see Interview: Coleborne and O'Hagan 2015).

When words are repurposed, they occupy a dangerous space in our shared speech. But this word 'madness' is important: it captures both the cultural artifact of mental breakdown from the past, and the present, lived-in worlds of those with mental illness conditions. It might productively allow us to own the problem of 'madness' collectively rather than to relegate it to the past, and to signal the histories of those who have been the subjects of psychiatry. 'Madness' is also used by historian Barbara Taylor, whose book *The Last Asylum: A Memoir of Madness in Our Times* was published in 2014. Taylor spent some of her thirties in the psychiatric wards of a famous nineteenth-century English institution, Colney Hatch, later known as Friern. She writes that 'the language of madness is controversial', but she goes on to use the word madness interchangeably with mental illness, partly to show its power as an everyday word that sums up much of her experience in her 'madness years' (Taylor 2015 [2014], xi). Taylor was discharged in 1992, after four years in and out of mental hospital wards. The institution itself closed the following year.

In their published and unpublished stories and oral narratives of institutions in the late twentieth century, we also come across the reflections
of former patients who tell of being able to wander around outside and
beyond the wards: 'Nice gardens and you could go out and walk around.
We weren't locked up during the daytime', said K, who was interviewed
about her short stay at one hospital following a breakdown (Coleborne
2012, 107). How, then, are the experiences of the institutionalised rendered in different contexts, and why has the clinical case record domi-
nated histories of mental health? Are there other ways inside the story of
madness? How do we talk and write about madness? What are the points
of tension and debate? Where are the silences?

There is a long tradition of what we might call 'mad writing' by those
who practised writing to escape from the asylum in their letters and
diaries (see Hornstein 2011; Sommer et al. 1998). Katharine Hodgkin
(2007) writes about the changing role for autobiographical accounts of
'madness'. 'From the eighteenth century onwards', explains Hodgkin,
'hospital treatment becomes the defining moment for mad autobiography' (195). This reminds us of the idea that madness emerged from the
institution itself: it is the result of this encounter between doctors and
the mad. By the twentieth century, that narrative was further character-
ised by newer forms of what Sigmund Freud and later exponents of therapeutic models called 'the talking cure'. Talking about madness is not so
new. But when considered as the motif or practice by historians, it has
the potential to shift the dominant narrative.

Different places have had their own established traditions of 'mad'
autobiography or famous figures who have written about mental illness.
There is a strong North American tradition of accounts by women
from the nineteenth and early twentieth centuries (see Geller and
Harris 1994). Mary Elene Wood's *The Writing on the Wall: Women's
Autobiography and the Asylum* (1994) focuses on the writings of women
such as American, Elizabeth Packard, who was 'made a prisoner' by her
husband of the asylum in Illinois in the 1860s and then wrote about
her experiences. Earlier examples of mad autobiography also exist, and
include the writings of early modern writer Hannah Allen.[1] Widowed
at 25, Hannah plunged into a 'deep melancholy'. Her memoir, *Satan
his Methods and Malice Baffled*, published in 1683, was an account of
her depression through stories of temptation, terrors, suicide attempts,
self-starvation and finally, recovery. Satan taunted her with apparitions,
strange lights, and forced her to blaspheme. She wrote on the walls with

scissors. She ingested opium, and smoked spiders in a pipe with tobacco. 'I soon after fell into a deep Despair, and my language and condition grew sadder than before. Now little to be heard from me, but lamenting my woeful state, and very sad and dreadful Expressions' (Allen 1683). It was reading Hannah's account that encouraged me to find ways to examine the history of mental breakdown, but in a new context: colonial Victoria, Australia.

There are many fictionalised accounts of the mad experience: famous novels, some of them iconic because of the status of their authors. Charlotte Perkins Gilman's story *The Yellow Wallpaper* (1892) or Sylvia Plath's *The Bell Jar* (1963) both evoke the painful worlds of internal struggle. New Zealand's tradition of 'mad' autobiography, witnessed primarily through the figure of writer Janet Frame (1924–2004) and her literary production, has at various times opened up discussion about mental health institutions in the twentieth-century past. Frame's experience is often a reference point for media discussions about institutions and psychiatric treatment. Her autobiographical account of growing up and experiencing mental breakdown, and being institutionalised, *An Angel at My Table*, was published in 1984 and was produced as a feature film (1990). Modern mental illness journeys, as Hodgkin (2007) suggests, have tended to be rendered as internalised journeys 'into the self' (196). They are defined by the use of diagnostic labels that offer hope to some, but which limit others, and such diagnoses can be difficult to escape.

Different historical periods provide specific possibilities, though some remain more silent than others. From the vantage point of 2019, as this book is published, we can now witness an array of possibilities in the story of madness over time. Throughout my career as a historian, I have found diverse ways to capture the worlds of madness and institutions, and to talk about madness. Starting with asylum records, such as patient cases, and along the way encountering museum collections of psychiatric objects, and now curious about the role of lived experience in the historical narrative, my own research journey has evolved as the practitioners in the field itself have also asked new questions of their subject, questions that are examined in turn in different chapters of this book.

My aim is that this book shares some of my reflections in an accessible manner. These include reflections about the way that archival 'cases' tell stories, and also suggest narratives of institutional experience, as set out in Chapter 2. The book also offers some insights into the institutional worlds occupied by patients or inmates in the past, in the era of large asylums and hospitals, including gender, power, class and spatial dynamics, and life in the worlds of institutions. The new histories provoked by institutional closures across western countries from the 1970s indicate new beginnings for the writing of history, both backwards and forwards in time. As Chapter 3 shows, these include public exhibition and display, and the work of museums to preserve institutional histories and to uncover hidden histories to larger audiences as educational tools for rethinking mental health in the present. The vital role played by families and communities in extra-institutional care discussed in Chapter 4 reveals the way that madness itself spills out and crosses over into institutional spaces, and is never fully 'contained' by institutional confinement. This chapter also points to more recent narratives of psychiatric survivors, mental health service-users, and those with lived experiences of madness from the places discussed in this book. Chapter 5 touches on the history of anti-psychiatry and presents a discussion about the politics of madness in public life. It describes the late-twentieth-century social movement around madness which enabled the psychiatric community to gain a new identity forged as survivors, consumers, service users, and advocates for humane and stigma-free mental health care. Finally, in Chapter 6, the book shows that more recent scholarly reflections on the theme of madness are signaling a profound shift in the historical and public imagination.

The most enduring form of historical writing about mental illness and hospitalisation has been a focus on the patient cases of psychiatric institutions of the nineteenth century, as Chapter 2 explains. Open and available to researchers, the archival records of these institutions afford researchers insights into the medical, clinical, social and cultural worlds of the institutionalised: worlds which included work and leisure time; practices of care and models of treatment; worlds which were permeable and from which patients and families came and went; and worlds formed inside regimes which labelled, categorised and ascribed identities to the 'insane' over time.

With access to all of these records, historians have been talking about 'patient-centred' histories of mental health since the 1980s. Yet histories that manage to achieve this are still rare, especially among histories focused on the more recent past. Scholars have reflected on whether our attempts to enter into the worlds of patients have been at all successful, even claiming that these histories have been neglected and underwritten (Bacopoulos-Viau and Fauvel 2016, 1–2). Canadian scholar-activists Megan Davies and Geoffrey Reaume, both based at York University in Toronto, produced a documentary, 'The Inmates are Running the Asylum: Stories from the MPA' (2012) about what happens when consumers of mental health services 'talk back' to the institutions and people who confined them in the twentieth century. The results of this agency—depending upon the national or local context—are challenging and sometimes surprising, as discussed in Chapter 5 of this book.

In setting out these ideas, my purpose is to establish a new scholarly context for such inquiry. Just how historians might navigate the waters between 'official' or biomedical accounts, and mental health service-user or consumer histories, results in a new politics of knowledge for the academic historian. Therefore, this book further maps out the tensions in this field and considers the variety of ways in which historians and other practitioners and writers, including filmmakers, might advance new ideas and discussion about mental health and its history. The book also engages with policy and government interventions. Being able to talk and tell stories of mental health is vital to recovery, well-being, and reconciliation. Sometimes this has taken place in the context of formal government inquiries, which have only partial success as a site of storytelling. Many other accounts of institutional abuses remain to be told. Still others are documented in film, patient writings such as pathography, and in creative forms.

Why Talk About Madness? presents innovative international research into mental health histories and extends our current knowledge about mental health histories into the twenty-first century. The book also moves the debate about writing histories of mental health forward in terms of the intellectual frameworks used by historians. Specifically, the book engages with interdisciplinary knowledge and considers historical writing in light of other disciplinary interventions. Building on existing scholarship in the fields of mental health, the title offers readers insights into the different worlds of mental illness, health, institutions, treatment, therapies, stories of the mind, of being out of mind, policies, notions of care and confinement, mental health recovery, advocacy and reactions to the experience of mental illness over time, such as institutional trauma. The collection also offers new ways of thinking about 'mad' history and writing, the question of the mental illness narrative over time and in context, about material cultures of illness and recovery, as well as the role of official inquiries as public events and narratives of intervention, as opposed to private stories and reflections on illness and depression. As I write, the national statistics for mental health problems in Australia reflect the global mental health crisis, with rising rates of suicide for young people identified by the WHO as the focus for the World Mental Health Day in October 2019.[2] Around twenty per cent of Australians experience a mental illness annually, with devastating results felt by local and national families, communities, workplaces and economies.

Finally, this book brings together the themes that have patterned my scholarly research into the asylum over a long period, allowing me to glance back at some of the central problems of evidence, gender in institutional contexts, sexed and raced bodies in colonial worlds, and the relevance of spatiality in the gendered institution. When madness was uncontained, it presented threat, challenge and opposition to the formation of theories of psychiatric knowledge and treatments. The bodies, behaviours and words of the mad in the past are valuable reminders of the difficulty inherent in mental illness conditions, but also of the deeply political idea of containment. My role as a historian is positioned and acknowledged here as being similar to that of an interpreter, making sense of the many different conversations on this topic, and from the vantage point of an observer and witness to historical ideas.

Notes

1. The earliest known work is by a woman named Margery Kempe (1438).
2. See https://www.who.int/mental_health/world-mental-health-day/2019/en/. Accessed 25 July 2019.

Suggested Reading

Allen, Hannah. 1683. *Satan his methods and malice baffled*. London: John Wallis.
Bacopoulos-Viau, Alexandra, and Aude Fauvel. 2016. The patient's turn: Roy Porter and psychiatry's tales, thirty years on. *Medical History* 60 (1): 1–18.
Beresford, Peter. 2014. Mad studies brings a voice of sanity to psychiatry. *Guardian*, October 7. https://www.theguardian.com/society/2014/oct/07/mad-studies-voice-of-sanity-psychiatry. Accessed October 2014.
Coleborne, Catharine. 2012. Patient journeys: Stories of mental health care from Tokanui to mental health services, 1930s to the 1980s. In *Changing times,*

changing places: From Tokanui to mental health services in the Waikato, 1910–2012, ed. Catharine Coleborne, 97–109. Hamilton: Half Court Press.

Coleborne, Catharine. 2015. *Insanity, identity and empire: Colonial institutional confinement in Australia and New Zealand, 1870–1910*. Manchester: Manchester University Press.

Coleborne, Catharine. 2017. An end to Bedlam? The enduring subject of madness in social and cultural history. *Social History* 42 (3): 420–429.

Coleborne, Catharine. 2018. Madness uncontained: A reflection. In *Containing madness: Gender and 'Psy' in institutional contexts*, eds Jennifer M. Kilty and Erin Dej, v–viii. Basingstoke: Palgrave.

Crossley, N. 1998. R. D. Laing and the British anti-psychiatry movement: A socio-cultural analysis. *Social Science and Medicine* 47 (7): 877–889.

Crossley, Michele L., and Nick Crossley. 2001. Patient voices, social movements and the habitus: how psychiatric survivors "speak out". *Social Science and Medicine* 52: 1477–1489.

Davies, Megan. 2012. The inmates are running the asylum: Stories from MPA. https://www.cinemapolitica.org/film/inmates-are-running-asylum-stories-mpa. Accessed July 2019.

Diamond, Paul. 2005. Whanau healing: How can Māori culture improve mental health? *The Listener*, September 24.

Durie, Mason. 1994. *Whaiora: Māori health development*. Auckland and New York: Oxford University Press.

Foucault, Michel. 1995. Madness, the absence of work, trans. Peter Stastny and Deniz Şengel. *Critical Inquiry* 21 (2): 290–298.

Frame, Janet. 1984. *An angel at my table: An autobiography, volume 2*. London: Women's Press.

Geller, Jeffrey L., and Maxine Harris. 1994. *Women of the asylum: Voices from behind the walls, 1840–1945*. New York, London, and Toronto: Anchor Books.

Gittins, Diana. 1998a. *Madness in its place: Narratives of Severalls Hospital, 1913–1997*. London and New York: Routledge.

Gittins, Diana. 1998b. Silences: The case of a psychiatric hospital. In *Narrative and genre*, eds Mary Chamberlain and Paul Thompson, 46–62. London and New York: Routledge.

Hodgkin, Katherine. 2007. *Madness in seventeenth-century autobiography*. Hampshire and New York: Palgrave.

Hornstein, Gail. 2011. A bibliography of first-person narratives of madness in English (5th Edition). https://static1.squarespace.com/static/599e-e1094c0dbff62a07fc13/t/59af1347dbe3974ceaa108b3/1355335733737/Bibliography+of+First-Person+Narratives+of+Madness+5th+edition.pdf. Accessed 1 August 2019.

Kritsotaki, Despo, Vicky Long, and Matthew Smith. eds. 2016. *Deinstitutionalisation and after: Post war psychiatry in the Western world.* Basingstoke: Palgrave.

LeFrançois, Brenda, Robert Menzies, and Geoffrey Reaume. eds. 2013. *Mad matters: A critical reader in Canadian mad studies.* Toronto: Toronto Canadian Scholars' Press.

McAllen, Jess. 2015. Shocking treatment. *Sunday Star Times,* January 25, Health Focus A9.

O'Hagan, Mary. 2014. *Madness made me: A memoir.* Wellington: Open Box.

O'Hagan, Mary. 2017. Madness in New Zealand. *Asylum: The Magazine for Democratic Psychiatry* 24 (2): 12–13.

Plath, Sylvia. 1966. *The bell jar.* London: Faber.

Porter, Roy. 1987. *A social history of madness: The world through the eyes of the insane.* New York: Weidenfeld & Nicolson.

Porter, Roy. 2002. *Madness: A brief history.* Oxford: Oxford University Press.

Sacks, Oliver. 2019 [2009]. The lost virtues of the asylum. In *Everything in its place,* 184–200. New York: Knopf; London: Picador.

Scull, Andrew. 2015. *Madness in civilization: A cultural history of insanity, from the Bible to Freud, from the madhouse to modern medicine.* Princeton, NJ: Princeton University Press.

Sommer, Robert, Jennifer S. Clifford, and John C. Norcross. 1998. A bibliography of mental patients' autobiographies: An update and classification system. *American Journal of Psychiatry* 155 (9) 1261–1264.

Szasz, Thomas. 1961. *The myth of mental illness: Foundations of a theory of personal conduct.* New York: Hoeber-Harper.

Taylor, Barbara. 2015 [2014]. *The last asylum: A memoir of madness in our times.* Chicago: University of Chicago Press.

Wood, Mary Elene. 1994. *The writing on the wall: Women's autobiography and the asylum.* Urbana: University of Illinois Press.

Interview: Catharine Coleborne and Mary O'Hagan, 21 May 2015, Wellington, New Zealand (1 hour and 35 minutes).

CHAPTER 2

Asylum Archives and Cases as Stories

Knowing madness—whether in utterances or writing, or through visual representation—has taken many forms. From the 'ship of fools' wood-cut of the 1500s, depicting the sequestration of lepers to a colony, to the array of mad actors in Hogarth's 'A Rake's Progress' paintings and engravings highlighting the world of 'Bedlam' and published in 1735, right through to the art and poetry by the mad themselves, dominant visual tropes and ideas about madness tend to shape our understandings of it. Even a brief survey of the covers of books on madness and the asy-lum reinforces the idea that although the 'patient' is the central repre-sentative figure in histories of madness, she or he is the most difficult to access. Images of the mad that are chosen to illustrate scholarly histo-ries are sometimes blurry, distorted, or are obviously the staged subjects of official asylum photography in its day. Researching at the Wellcome Library in the 1990s, I found a case from Hanwell Asylum, Middlesex: a young woman inmate photographed for the institutional record in the 1880s, held back by asylum staff to capture her grimace and surly gaze. In the nineteenth century, photography was a new technology of surveil-lance and objectification in medicine. Yet such photographs also offer us the possibility of finding the records of 'real people and their suffering', to paraphrase Barbara Brookes (2011, 31). They also take us beyond the words and framings of the clinical narrative and offer insight into 'indi-vidual subjects' (Du Plessis 2015, 94–95).

Rendering the experience of madness—embodied, visceral and men-tal—is a complicated process for historians and other scholars. It has

© The Author(s) 2020
C. Coleborne, *Why Talk About Madness?* Mental Health in Historical
Perspective, https://doi.org/10.1007/978-3-030-21096-0_2

been heavily mediated and shaped by the availability of accounts of madness. Trying to represent madness is now even viewed as a form of voyeurism in some quarters. Sander Gilman broke new ground in his work *Seeing the Insane* (1982), which in conceptual terms, advanced similar ideas to those of Foucault, arguing that visual representations of madness produced meanings about mental illness over time. More than this, Gilman's suggestion that madness was 'othered' much like ethnic difference, leading to labelling and exclusion, proved powerful in an emerging discussion about the stereotyping of people suffering with mental illness conditions.

Putting madness experiences into her own words, Mary O'Hagan suggested that:

> Well, they are experiences that affect your ... they affect everything. They affect your intellect, they affect your sensory experiences, your sense of having free will. They affect you physically, they affect your relationships. And they're kind of extreme, overwhelming states of mind that affect all those things. (Interview Coleborne and O'Hagan 2015)

Historians have consistently found it difficult to translate such experiences into writing. Traditional historical research methods also strain against the very notion of 'experience', and even practitioners of oral history methodologies, keen to justify their work, tend to shy away from the idea of presenting undiluted narrative accounts of experience without analysing their contents; yet at the same time such intellectual processes can be very powerful, and add value to oral accounts. Interdisciplinary work offers more possibilities: using art, drama and digital communication to represent madness would extend historians and allow new ways of seeing madness. These points are important because this chapter suggests that the available histories of madness fall short in many respects. At the same time, historians have been at the forefront of trying to understand it at all, and their work should be understood more widely as vital to our collective understandings of mental health.

By the early twenty first century, the well-established mode of writing institutional histories of madness of the long nineteenth century has involved the sampling of available patient case notes from archival collections, mostly in national and provincial repositories. Such data provides material for the analysis of patient populations, patterns of admission and discharge, diagnoses and treatments, as well as insights into institutional practices affecting people with mental illness conditions. Canadian historian David Wright has traced the vast body of historical scholarship, calling it an 'archipelago' of findings about this network of asylums and its common features across many national boundaries, also drawing attention to the highly ambiguous nature of institutions and their objectives over time (Wright 2018). What *was* the institution, but more importantly for this book, what impact did it have on people?

One of the most interesting examples of these histories is *Remembrance of Patients Past* (2009) by Canadian academic, Geoffrey Reaume, an advocate of mad peoples' histories from the insider perspective. Reaume was drawn to this material in part because of his own experience of hospitalisation in Ontario institutions in the 1970s. His book opens with the words of a patient at the Toronto hospital for the insane, and an image of the patient. Reaume (2009) writes that he aims to 'present inmates in mental institutions as individual human beings who deserve to be understood on their own terms as *people*' (original emphasis, 5). Everything in this scholarly account points to the centrality of the patient experience—of admission, of work therapies, of routine, of leisure time, of interactions with others, and of getting out of the asylum. Where Reaume's work is distinctive is in the way he interprets diagnoses through a critical reading of social context. 'Distress', he writes, 'had to do with the depredations brought on by poverty, social isolation, loss of status and income, and abuse from people in positions of power' (Reaume 2009, 53).

Like this work, many historians in the post-1970s social history boom have written accounts of mental illness and the asylum through similar prisms of social, cultural and political contexts to position and understand madness in place and time. North American historians paved the way for others keen to understand new dimensions in the institutional populations of large asylums, include Richard W. Fox, whose study of over one thousand cases of asylum inmates in 1870s–1930 California was a landmark in the field (1979). Gerald Grob's work has been especially influential; he wrote about mental illness and society, and he raised questions about social difference and the fear of otherness in new societies and their populations because of the spectre of madness (see Grob 1966; 1983). Grob's *The Mad Among Us* (1994) appealed to me as a scholar starting out because of his framing of the asylum as an 'invention': like other historians and sociologists, Grob's interpretation of the institution was that it filled the social needs created by rapid urbanisation and industrialisation of post-1800 America (Grob 1994, 23–25). These histories of early North American asylums were important because it was a newer society in the shadow of competing imperial interests, with a longer history of adaptation of British models of law, medicine and its institutions. Studies of specific institutions, their populations, comparisons between places, gender, class, ethnicity, diagnoses, the impact of immigration, and the formation of asylums in the colonised worlds of India, South Africa, Canada, Fiji, Australia, New Zealand, the Caribbean and a range of African countries, now demonstrate the sheer scale of spread of psychiatry and its practices from the British world to these newer societies and places from the mid-1800s to the mid-twentieth century. The histories of asylums and peoples in all of these sites add to the global history of what it has meant to be mad over time.

How these worlds differed across places is also important, and the nuances of institutional care across the British world are part of this history. These institutional spaces produced regimes and cultures of patient movement, patterns of life, and boundaries and restraints, both physical and mental. There are many examples of these asylum spaces: for example, the typically small 'airing yards' for inmates to pace; the introduction of garden environments; and the use of walls, corridors and wards for the herding of patients by the twentieth century. Gender was an early form of difference used to organise asylum spaces. Separating women and men into different wards was part of the function of the reformative asylum by the middle of the nineteenth century, with authorities intent on moral therapies including gendered forms of labour and religious worship; the pinnacle of the therapeutic approach was allowing patients who were deemed well enough to attend asylum balls and outings where they would mix with members of the public. Ethnicity became another form of difference used to create spaces inside institutions. South African historians, and historians interested in colonial India, write about the practice of separating out populations into different institutional spaces. India's asylums for the insane catered to different populations; 'natives' were sent to one type of institution, while the 'European insane' were treated separately (Porter and Wright, eds 2003; Mills 2003; Ernst 1991).

The institutions all over the world quickly became somewhat failed experiments, with overcrowding, violence, poverty, illness and disease turning asylums into bleak places of despair, subject to inquiries and legal complaints. New scholarship revisits these 'cultures of madness', showing that the deep wrestling with these histories remains important for our own societies (Dunk 2019). Writing about the historical geographies of asylum in Scotland and England, Hester Parr and Chris Philo and colleagues have explored the idea of madness in place (see Parr and Philo 1995).[1] Material cultures of past institutions offer new possibilities to interpret the lives of people in these spaces. Linnea Kuglitsch is examining the archaeology of psychiatric institutions and highlighting the emotions embedded in material objects, describing this as a 'distinct dataset' of realities and lived experiences, because physical artefacts also enter the historical record (Kuglitsch 2018). These exciting methodologies promise to challenge the older forms of knowledge-making based in clinical records, allowing, as she says, the 'tender remembrances' of the mad to be included as evidence of lived experiences of madness inside places and environments of the past.

Roy Porter's invitation to write history from 'the patient's view' (see Porter 1985) inspired generations of scholars in the social histories of health and medicine. The histories of madness, insanity and the asylum proved to be a rich source of patients' records, with one major problem: these clinical and administrative records were *produced about* confined individuals and present challenges for historians wanting firsthand accounts of what it means to be 'mad'. Methods of reading both along and against 'the grain' of archival sources assist scholars to understand the people and points of view inside these case histories (Coleborne 2010, 151). Therefore, in my own estimation, these are not 'lost lives' as Sally Swartz has suggested (Swartz 1999, 152–158). By supplementing cases with patient and family letters, patients' depositions to formal inquiries, patient testimony and writings, as well as other forms of firsthand accounts by the institutionalised, historians can help to round out the picture, and add meaningful dimensions to the depiction of institutionalised peoples. As Reaume put it, 'family and community responses' to madness could be 'intertwined with prejudice and misunderstanding' (Reaume 2009, 208).

Without doubt, the lives of the mad in these records constitute a rich trove for researchers who can obtain reasonably open access to institutional archives. Genealogists, for example, find family members in the patient casebooks, aided by indexes and matching birth, death and marriage records, as well as shipping records when migration is part of the history. The linking of people in these various official records of population is an immensely satisfying activity: the finding of a person in the asylum can be a surprise and is often the missing piece of a jigsaw of family history. It can point, too, to stories of pain, heredity, and anxiety about generational mental health.

Institutional archival populations of the eighteenth and nineteenth centuries present opportunities to reflect on patients' experiences both at home and inside the asylums. The interventions of the historian into that archive can tell us about the way institutional populations of the mad were gendered; and how the very poor tended to be caught in a net of welfare and social institutions. For instance, in her study of gender and class in English asylums at the end of the nineteenth century, Louise Hide follows other historians in her casting of the institution as a place where populations of the mad were 'made' through these labels (Hide 2014, 14–39). My own study of the institutions across the Australasian colonies argues that the 'populations and processes of social institutions' tell us about societies in formation, making use of the social categories of class, gender, ethnicity, age and sexuality (Coleborne 2015, 2).

Whether women were more mad than men is a question that drove much research into the patterns of institutional committal (Showalter 1987; Busfield 1996; Lunbeck 1994). In my writing about women as patients in colonial asylums in Australia, we can interpret the work of bodies inside institutional spaces, and their traces in the material cultures of place, as evidence of institutional constraints and resistance (Coleborne 2007). Within the spaces of the asylum, female patients could challenge and sometimes confound asylum methods of cure. This resistance was found in the rejection of force-feeding or hydrotherapies, visible reactions to official institutional photography, the world of interactions between inmates and attendants and medical personnel, and in the art of escape.

The overwhelming numbers of labouring men in asylums of the nineteenth-century highlight the way industrialisation and urbanisation in both the old and new countries of the world forced mobility, social dislocation, problems of health and nutrition, as well as family breakdown and poverty, all of which contributed to a growth in asylum populations. Men confronted a world of technological change; accounts of delusions in the patient record in the nineteenth century show a preoccupation with communications technologies, such as sound or the telegraph (Coleborne 2015, 125).

For indigenous peoples in Australia, New Zealand and Canada, asylums became places of cultural disorientation and separation.

In Australia, an early study of Aboriginal insane conducted by asylum superintendent Frederic Norton Manning offers a rare glimpse of the treatment of indigenous peoples in early Sydney (see Coleborne 2010, 39). The biographical account of Tarra Bobby, an Aboriginal man in colonial Victoria, tells us more about these encounters between European social, legal and medical institutions (Attwood 1987).

In Auckland, New Zealand, few Māori peoples were confined at Te Whau, but those who were found themselves inside a white European institutional culture, and similarly exhibited *mate Māori* or cultural alienation (Burke and Coleborne 2011, 295); many died of tuberculosis following their committal. Robert Menzies and Ted Palys portray the aboriginal patients of British Columbia as 'turbulent spirits' (Menzies and Palys 2006, 149). They recount the cases of men like Charley Wolverine, who became 'dull and seclusive' in the 1940s after hospitalisation.

As historians write about large data—the vast number of patient cases in the record—critical tensions emerge between the micro-histories of individual lives, and the overarching narrative of these institutions and their mobile populations. A few examples of focusing on individual stories offer other ways of entering more deeply into the record and extrapolating rich 'genealogies of the intimate' (Wilbraham 2014, 185). Using one life, one story, one person, can be an effective way to fan out and reach into the experiences of family members or migration stories, examining how one person's encounter with the asylum was part of a much larger family narrative. The 'partial truths' of the patient record are then made more obvious (Wilbraham 2014, 184). Patient case records can be viewed as one 'genre' in the array of textual representations of madness. As I suggest in my own work about colonial asylums in Victoria, Australia, the patient case file did not have a neat narrative; its subjects were 'shifting', hard to pin down, and they refused, in some instances, the attempts at categorisation or classification made so popular by the nineteenth-century age of data collection (Coleborne 2007, 57–79).

What kinds of stories *are* these? Scull argued in his reflective *The Insanity of Place/The Place of Insanity* (2006) that there are dangers in 'romanticising' madness when telling the stories of the insane. Worried about the sheer difficulty of accessing patients' own words through medical records, and about the ways, these are the result of an imbalance of power, his overarching concern with attempts to consider these narratives is with the concept of knowledge: the capacity to know and understand a mediated experience (51). He acknowledges the fine work of those historians who have sought to examine the families and the agency and purpose of those advocating for the mad, particularly the important work of David Wright and others writing in the late 1990s on that theme in parts of Britain (Wright 1997; 1998).

Other kinds of accounts can add to the larger narrative of the patient. Allan Ingram's study, *The Madhouse of Language* (1991) offers an analysis of accounts from the eighteenth century and shows how questions of our very accessibility to experience have defined the responses to writing by those experiencing madness. In the modern era, the stories of those with lived experience of mental illness can also be difficult to obtain. Writing by sufferers of mental illness does not take the form of the classic illness narrative or pathography, usually written by a survivor of a life-threatening illness who wins a battle against a disease. Instead, mental illness presents problems of cycles of illness, treatment, recovery and relapse (Campion 2009, 22). What is common among written accounts of hospitalisation is a sense of identity under threat, something exacerbated by the legal confinement of mentally ill persons inside institutional spaces. These feelings of powerlessness remind us of the loss of liberty wrought by the tragedy of mental illness. In much writing, there is a blurring of asylum as sanctuary and asylum as custodial, a problem which has dogged institutions for mental health since the nineteenth century.

Most academic histories now include patient case records as evidence, as well as a focus on how to make sense of these cases. As a historian of psychiatry, mental institutions and the 'mad' in Apartheid South Africa, Tiffany Fawn Jones asserts, psychiatric practices were so 'imposing' that their history cannot be comprehended without patients' perspectives (Jones 2012, 58). Jones writes interestingly of the various challenges facing historians when they attempt to write histories of psychiatry from the 'patient-centred' point of view. The largest impediment to such a project, she suggests, is that patients' narratives are not homogenous (59). As well as this, many official sources including patient records and letters have been lost, destroyed, censored, and were clearly repressive of inmates' voices; the institutionalised were stigmatised, and their very experiences embody a lack of privacy for patients to articulate their worlds at all (58–59).

Yet in all of this effort to enter the worlds of madness through its records, as Sally Swartz writes, 'where is the madness represented?' (Swartz 2018, 297). Narratives of the mad derived from patient records do not always give us this type of powerful insight into being mad, but they can tell us different things about institutions. Poignant stories emerged from a project to write a collaborative history of a New Zealand institution (see Coleborne and the Waikato Mental Health History Group 2012, 100–103), and access was granted to view selected patient files from the 1930s to the 1960s. Among these cases was an example of a young woman with postpartum mania in the 1930s, hospitalised following childbirth.[2] Doctors speculated that childbirth had exacerbated her condition. They also worried about her intellectual capacity, and by implication, her capacity for parenting. Reading her notes, we find more about the social aspects of this woman's experiences. Her family was under economic stress by the later 1930s. By her second admission in July 1936, she was aged in her early 30s with a four-year-old child, and was living apart from her parents and siblings, whose situation was one of extreme poverty. Her husband was now an unemployed farmer; he had declared himself unable to care for her during periods of mental illness. Confused, and suffering from delusions, this woman spent six months in the psychiatric hospital before her discharge.[3] She maintained her dignity inside the hospital and kept herself busy with a knitting bag. By the early 1950s, when she again spent time at the same institution, the property she brought with her was itemised in two lists. Among the everyday items—suitcase, attaché case, dresses, cardigans, stockings and so on—was a fur stole, and a pair of kid gloves. Other belongings were listed too: her wedding ring, keys, savings book, insurance policy, birth and marriage certificates, and sent to the Public Trustee in August 1950 as part of her estate kept under protection during her period of hospitalisation.[4] These practices imply that patients were now 'protected' by the State during periods of mental illness. However, families did not abandon their loved ones. They wrote to doctors, and together, navigated the typical arc of admission, probation and discharge, and readmission.

Another woman's journeys to Tokanui, around the same time, illustrates the dimensions of class difference and ethnicity in the experience of mental illness and institutionalisation. A Māori woman, diagnosed as schizophrenic, had multiple admissions to Tokanui from 1943 to 1959, but the files indicate no family visits to her took place. She was placed in solitary confinement for long periods of time in 1959. In August, September and November her hours of solitary confinement averaged around ten per day and amounted to more than 70 hours a week in some weeks. Unlike some other women, she came with very few belongings. In 1959, she brought with her a dressing gown, a rug, a cotton cardigan, a torn petticoat (described as 'rags') and one singlet. Her physical health was in poor shape: she was bruised, had several weeping skin sores, and was regularly treated with penicillin; she was poorly nourished. Sadly, the record reveals that she had placed her baby and other people in harmful and violent situations. She had also come into contact with the police, trying to buy beer from them in her home town of Huntly. She and members of her family were described as illiterate, unable to manage their affairs, and were living out cyclic family situations of ill-health. Her daughter became a mental health patient, aged 22.[5]

The stories found inside the clinical case notes tell us about a few aspects of patients' lives both inside and outside the institution. For example, poverty, ethnicity and social class shaped family experiences of mental illness, with committals viewed throughout the medical notes as an extension of patients' social situations in impoverished families and communities. Some patients were then treated more directly as a violent and difficult patient in physical terms, while others received periodic, and what was perceived to be reasonably effective, electro-convulsive therapy (ECT). There were families who tried hard to maintain contact with institutional authorities, going to the trouble of sending patients clothing, only to find their son or daughter dressed 'shabbily' for a visit home. Patients either brought few items with them, or, despite their family's situations, came with many pieces of clothing, and with things to do. All of these stories point to mental illness as an experience which can demolish families and tear apart the lives of individuals, however useful the periods of institutional care.

While partial and episodic, these case notes provide glimpses of madness as an experience (Coleborne 2017). To return to the ideas of Sally Swartz (1999), we can suggest that the overall effect of the creation of these short narratives is often—despite our own compassionate tone as historians—distancing. The power relations embedded in the institutional record, and its archive, present challenges for those of us trying to represent past voices. These are case studies, drawn from a record of institutional confinement. What happens if we change and shift the authorial position? What new power relations does it set up? And what is it, exactly, that such accounts can tell us?

More recently, and as mental health service-user and advocacy communities increasingly focus on the rights of those people with lived experiences of mental illness, these scholarly and historical accounts of patients and the asylum—using language derived from institutional clinical materials—can seem exploitative to some audiences. The ethics of using such case materials has also been under scrutiny. Debates about using patient case materials, and referring to individuals by name, include the reflections of researchers about our continued access to archival sources such as patient cases, and the question of openness and visibility of people who lived in the institutions and whose stories deserve to be told and understood (see Garton 2000, 45; Wright and Saucier 2012, 77).

These accounts of institutional archives, patient cases, the stories of madness, the interventions of the mad and their supporters, all help us to position the role of the narrative of madness in the wider narrative of mental health history. Despite emerging ethical concerns about access to institutional records, the rich repository of research methods and accounts created by historians suggest that these cases might be read as early examples of the power of personal storytelling in the context of institutional regimes. It is the case, as Erika Dyck and Alex Deighton suggest, that patients 'left their marks' on the asylum (Dyck and Deighton 2017, 8). By the late twentieth century, the outspoken voices of those in the mental health consumer movement echo earlier forms of speech from inside the asylum. At the same time, they provide a new set of narratives for the histories of madness. In earlier periods, the institution's immense control over the lives of people—and its capacity to frame narratives and patient cases—shows that change over time in the treatment, care and understanding of madness was slow. Much of this is due to the institutional regimes themselves: the uses of space that shaped the everyday experience of madness, as well as the powerful work of memories of place in creating a sense of the asylum long after it was closed.

NOTES

1. Exciting projects building on Philo's published works are mentioned here: https://asylumspaces.wordpress.com/2014/06/26/introducing-prof-chris-philo/. Accessed 31 July 2019.
2. Archives New Zealand (ANZ), YCBG (Tokanui Hospital Patient Files) 5904, Box 40, 1074-1091 (1931–32). For the later periods of time spent at Tokanui, see subsequent references.

3. YCGB 5904, Box 60, 1468-1491 (1936).
4. YCBG 5904, Box 185, 3408-3428 (1950).
5. YCBG 5905, Box 82, 938-950, c. 1968.

SUGGESTED READINGS

Attwood, Bain. 1987. Tarra Bobby, a Brataualung man. *Aboriginal History* 11 (1–2): 41–57.

Brookes, Barbara. 2011. Pictures of people, pictures of places: Photography and the asylum. In *Exhibiting madness in museums: Remembering psychiatry through collections and display*, eds Catharine Coleborne and Dolly MacKinnon, 30–47. New York: Routledge.

Burke, Lorelle, and Catharine Coleborne. 2011. Insanity and ethnicity in New Zealand: Māori encounters with the Auckland Mental Hospital, 1860–1900. *History of Psychiatry* 22 (3): 285–301.

Busfield, Joan. 1996. *Men, women, and madness: Understanding gender and mental disorder.* London: Macmillan Press.

Campion, Michelle. 2009. Narratives from the mind's eye: The significance of mental health pathography in New Zealand, 1980–2008. PhD thesis, University of Waikato, New Zealand.

Coleborne, Catharine. 2007. *Reading 'madness': Gender and difference in the colonial asylum in Victoria, Australia, 1848–1880.* Perth, WA: Network Books.

Coleborne, Catharine. 2010. *Madness in the family: Insanity and institutions in the Australasian colonial world, 1860–1914.* Basingstoke, Hampshire and New York: Palgrave Macmillan.

Coleborne, Catharine. 2015. *Insanity, identity and Empire: Colonial institutional confinement in Australia and New Zealand, 1870–1910.* Manchester: Manchester University Press.

Coleborne, Catharine, and the Waikato Mental Health History Group, eds. 2012. *Changing times, changing places: From Tokanui Hospital to mental health services in the Waikato, 1910–2012.* Hamilton, NZ: Half Court Press.

Coleborne, Catharine. 2017. Institutional case files. In *Sources and methods in histories of colonialism: Approaching the imperial archive*, eds Kirsty Reid and Fiona Paisley, 113–128. London and New York: Routledge.

Dunk, James. 2019. *Bedlam at Botany Bay.* Sydney, NSW: NewSouth Publishing.

Du Plessis, Rory. 2015. Beyond a clinical narrative: Casebook photographs from the Grahamstown Lunatic Asylum, c. 1890s. *Critical Arts: South-North Cultural and Media Studies* 29 (1): 88–103.

Dyck, Erika, and Alex Deighton. 2017. *Managing madness: Weyburn mental hospital and the transformation of psychiatric care in Canada.* Winnipeg, Canada: University of Manitoba Press.

Ernst, Waltraud. 1991. *Mad tales from the Raj: The European insane in British India, 1800–1858.* London and New York: Routledge.

Fox, Richard W. 1979. *So far disordered in mind: Insanity in California, 1870–1930.* Berkeley: University of California Press.

Garton, Stephen. 2000. Shut off from the source: A national obsession with privacy has led to fears for the future of Australian social history. *Australian,* November 22. http://www.asap.unimelb.edu.au/asa//aus-archivists/msg00470.html. Accessed 1 August 2019.

Gilman, Sander. 1982. *Seeing the insane: A cultural history of madness and art in the Western world.* New York and Chichester: Wiley/Brunner-Mazel.

Grob, Gerald N. 1966. *The state and the mentally ill: A history of Worcester State Hospital in Massachusetts, 1830–1920.* Chapel Hill: University of North Carolina Press.

Grob, Gerald N. 1983. *Mental illness and American society, 1875–1940.* Princeton, NJ: Princeton University Press.

Grob, Gerald N. 1994. *The mad among us: A history of the care of America's mentally ill.* Cambridge, MA and London: Harvard University Press.

Hide, Louise. 2014. *Gender and class in English asylums, 1890–1914.* London: Palgrave Macmillan UK.

Jones, Tiffany Fawn. 2012. *Psychiatry, mental institutions, and the mad in apartheid South Africa.* New York and London: Routledge.

Kuglitsch, Linnea. 2018. "Kindly hearts and tender hands": Exploring the asylum and patient narratives through the archaeological record. Society for the Social History of Medicine Conference, Liverpool, UK, 11–13 July.

Lunbeck, Elizabeth. 1994. *The psychiatric persuasion: Knowledge, gender, and power in modern America.* Princeton, NJ: Princeton University Press.

Menzies, Bob, and Ted Palys. 2006. Turbulent spirits: Aboriginal patients in the British Columbia psychiatric system, 1879–1950. In *Mental health and Canadian society: Historical perspectives,* eds James E. Moran and David Wright, 149–175. Montreal and Kingston, London, Ithaca: McGill-Queen's University Press.

Mills, James. 2003. *Cannabis Britannica: Empire, trade and prohibition, 1800–1928.* Oxford and New York: Oxford University Press.

Parr, Hester, and Chris Philo. 1995. Mapping mad identities. In *Mapping the subject: Geographies of cultural transformation,* eds Steve Pile and N. J. Thrift, 199–225. London and New York: Routledge.

Porter, Roy. 1985. The patient's view: Doing medical history from below. *Theory and Society* 14 (2): 175–198.

Porter, Roy, and David Wright, eds. 2003. *The confinement of the insane: International perspectives, 1800–1965.* Cambridge, UK and New York: Cambridge University Press.

Reaume, Geoffrey. 2009. *Remembrance of patients past: Patient life at the Toronto Hospital for the insane, 1870–1940*. Toronto, ON: University of Toronto Press.

Showalter, Elaine. 1987. *The female malady: Women, madness and English culture 1830–1980*. London: Virago.

Swartz, Sally. 1999. Lost lives: Gender, history and mental illness in the Cape, 1891–1910. *Feminism and Psychology* 9 (2): 152–158.

Swartz, Sally. 2018. Asylum case records: Fact and fiction. *Rethinking History* 22 (2): 289–301.

Wilbraham, Lindy. 2014. Reconstructing Harry: A genealogical study of a colonial family 'inside' and 'outside' the Grahamstown asylum, 1888–1918. *Medical History* 58 (2): 166–187.

Wright, David. 1997. Getting out of the asylum: Understanding the confinement of the insane in the nineteenth century. *Social History of Medicine* 10 (1): 137–155.

Wright, David. 1998. Family strategies and the institutional confinement of idiots in Victorian England. *Journal of Family History* 23: 189–208.

Wright, David. 2018. The great confinement revisited: What have we learned after 40 years of asylum studies? Society for the Social History of Medicine Conference, 11–13 July.

Wright, David, and Renee Saucier. 2012. Madness in the archives: Anonymity, ethics, and mental health history research. *Journal of the Canadian Historical Association* 23 (2): 65–90.

Interview: Catharine Coleborne and Mary O'Hagan, 21 May 2015, Wellington, New Zealand (1 hour and 35 minutes).

CHAPTER 3

The Asylum and Its Afterlife

Psychiatric institutions articulated and arranged ideas about madness. The worlds inside the psychiatric institutions of the nineteenth century and into the twentieth century were sharply delineated spaces, defined by walls, gates, passageways, wards, and corridors. These places and spaces of madness were as much about gender, control and order as they were sanitation and institutional mental hygiene. As Andrew Scull put it, the large asylums of history 'organised' madness. They were, in his estimation, like 'museums'—they collected and classified forms of mental illness—and because of the pressures created by overcrowding, they tended to be more custodial than curative (Scull 1979). Scull refined his ideas about institutions over time, reprising earlier comments about asylums in his later work *The Most Solitary of Afflictions*, a study that placed institutions into a wider social context (1993).

Asylums were supposed to be places of refuge, quiet and safety. Over time they acquired a multitude of meanings, from 'human and creative retreats' to places of disappointment in the public imagination, with dark Victorian histories (Scull 1996, 7–9). As Chapter 4 goes on to describe, it was the opening up of the asylum in the twentieth century that made new ideas about asylum possible from the points of view of those who had lived in and with the institution; as a 'new dialogue between sanity and madness' emerged, and new concepts of the space itself could be articulated (Wallcraft 1996, 186). Erving Goffman's idea of the 'total institution' was a powerful intervention in the 1960s made at a time when these institutional walls were being pulled down—both

© The Author(s) 2020   29
C. Coleborne, *Why Talk About Madness?* Mental Health in Historical
Perspective, https://doi.org/10.1007/978-3-030-21096-0_3

metaphorically and actually—by a movement concerned with exposing the institutional violence of psychiatry and its treatments. Goffman observed the spatiality of the institution, its routines, practices and regimes of power and social relations; his idea of 'total institution' and the 'social establishment' described the worlds shaping the behaviours of all inside it including medical and nursing staff (Goffman 1961).

Institutions have garnered their own identities in communities, places, and landscapes over time. Slang terms (often demeaning and derogatory) for the madhouse take on mythical status in the minds of people who have grown up in their midst, only faintly aware of their function. Institutions become part of the stories of places, too, and following institutional closures, begin to assume the status of 'built heritage'. Scull's 'museums of madness' was a metaphor for asylum populations, but also had the effects of portraying asylums as static monuments to ideas about insanity at a specific time (1979). Though historical research shows that some of these institutions were far more permeable than previously imagined, with closure, many asylums really did become 'museums'— vacant sites whose crumbling edifices retained dark memories etched into their interior walls and corners. For example, the former 'Bedlam' is now the Imperial War Museum in London. Some asylums, including Kew Metropolitan Asylum in Victoria, Australia, were repurposed as apartments, and others as university campuses. In a few examples, communities have created 'friends' groups and established museum spaces to share histories and knowledge about nursing and mental health (see Coleborne 2003). The 'adaptive re-use' of former asylums has been the subject of debate, scholarship and cultural heritage policy (Osborne 2003). The 'archaeological footprint' of institutions can tell us more about the worlds of the mad: the many lost trinkets, keepsakes and items never passed to families following the deaths of asylum inmates constitute a different material archive of memories of madness (Kuglitsch 2018).

These institutional worlds therefore had considerable afterlife status well into the late twentieth and twenty-first centuries, living on through public art projects, built heritage and museum collections and exhibitions. Institutional closures, then, promoted new forms of historical representation of madness, including writing about asylums as places with local and institutional histories. The memories and stories of staff and workers inside institutions are part of this larger narrative. The 'tall tales' of these institutions circulating in the popular imagination were also prevalent by the latter part of the twentieth century. All of this cultural production tells us that the role of institutions to create stories of madness—indeed, to stimulate these—means that institutional closures were dramatic and significant for communities and individuals.

How did this happen? As institutional closures happened, they signaled what I call a rupture in the narrative of mental health histories. This rupture, as the word suggests, was in fact a violent change to the status quo: institutions that had existed as the main forms and places of care and treatment of those with mental illness were being *shut down*, and people who lived and worked inside these places were being *moved out*. Yet although rupture means sudden, and complete, break, the process of deinstitutionalisation could be perceived from the outside as being more gradual. It was also an uneven process, as historians show (Kritsotaki et al. 2016, 5) and a 'confusing, complicated process' for communities (Burge 2015, 286). Yet rupture still provides a sense of the stark shift that took place for those who had lived inside one paradigm for mental health and who would now face a new way of thinking about the future.

Rupture is also a useful term because deinstitutionalisation was a change that propelled new ways of talking about the problems associated with mental illness as madness became more visible in communities, instead of being shut away inside institutions. Institutional closures created a demonstrable gap between the relative 'silence' around mental illness, and the possibility of 'talk' about mental illness and its treatments. These processes of change therefore created the conditions for the greater visibility of what had been an emerging public dissent about the role of the mental health institution during the 1950s and 1960s. Rupture, then, helps us to express the full meaning of this changing historical narrative. The 'inside' was now 'outside'; institutional closures created aggressive changes in the communication of mental illness in public, changes in the talk about it, and it forced new audiences to listen to stories of mental breakdown. These new beginnings for mental health talk and dissent offer up powerful examples of history in action.

This narrative of institutional closures is a collective story: when whole institutions closed, institutional populations were transferred from the confines of institutions and into the wider communities around them, sometimes enabled by community support, and at other times, without any structural supports at all. It is, then, a story and history that has many dimensions: it is local, affecting local communities and economies, and it is also global, a transnational history of changes in the way we have thought about mental health and institutions. This is what makes the story of psychiatric care in the twentieth century ripe for reinvestigation both across national boundaries, and in ways that invite new modes of seeing and understanding the historical traces of mental illness in space and time.

We have reminders of the occupation of the now empty and abandoned spaces of mental hospitals in the late twentieth century found in patient graffiti, objects and furniture, and in the memories and stories of hospitalisation. Yet it is difficult to understand spaces historically, to record and understand their meanings for people who occupied them (McGeachan 2017, 59). In a series of photographic images of psychiatric hospitals in New Zealand, Clare Goodwin (2004) portrays the 'shadows and silences' in the empty spaces of formerly bustling and inhabited spaces. These images remind us of the functions of these spaces for former residents. The view from a window of tall grass outside serves as a reminder of one institution's abandonment. In another image, the depiction of derelict bathtubs tells the story of a collective loss of privacy and a forced institutional intimacy of patients. These are powerful images that also tell a story of the traces of life of many people who occupied the spaces of the hospital. Other photographs of institutions linger over corridors, windows, the security which kept some in, and others out. Sacks writes about Christopher Payne's book *Asylum*, which also offers 'elegiac' imagery of former institutions in their desolate and abandoned states (Sacks 2019, 192–193).

By contrast, the 'Mad Love' installation in the Wellcome Exhibition 'Bedlam: The Asylum and Beyond' (September 2016–January 2017) was a utopian, hopeful work of art. The imaginary 'designer asylum' created by people with lived experience of mental illness showed both an interior and exterior world of spaces for recovery based on sensory perceptual concepts. Animals, space for contemplation, social and private spaces, as well as viewpoints and areas to roam, all define this world of madness. It is a welcoming space—and in its challenge to exhibition visitors, it asked just how we all occupy a world of mental health.

There is growing evidence that the post-institutional era presents historians with new sources to tell these stories. The historical process of deinstitutionalisation left us with residue and remains; with the kinds of memories that are both material and ephemeral. The material cultures of institutions, the personal effects of people who experienced institutions, and the visual record of institutional spaces, all provide us with a strong set of reminders of the worlds inside institutions, as the previous chapter described. Here, I want to focus on how these reminders have been used in the rewriting of mental health history through visual display, exhibition, museum collections and their public outreach and impact. These elements have been instrumental to the work of the mad movement: to the public imaginary and concept of madness and its meanings over time.

The idea of the 'still-present' past is taken from an exhibition at the Adam Art Gallery at the University of Victoria, Wellington, in New Zealand, in 2005.[1] The phrase evokes in a very powerful way the problem of talking about madness and institutions close to their own historical time, especially for those people with lived experiences of the institutions. In England, historian Barbara Taylor's *The Last Asylum: A Memoir in Our Times* (2015 [2014]) also points to this tension and the almost electric current of anxiety inherent to such closures for individuals, as well as for institutional groups. Taylor describes being close to the process of moving in and out of particular kinds of institutions, and into the 'halfway' space of supervised community care. At times she was terrified by the openness of it, but she was also able to observe and witness it as it happened, making her insights valuable in the context of the history of deinstitutionalisation (Taylor 2015 [2014], 188–196).

Museums have always played a role in the creation of public memory as social, cultural, and political institutions. In the present, museums are more than repositories, archives, or basement shelves and temperature-controlled rooms for manuscripts, artworks or objects. As expert museologists, historians, and museum curators all know, the contemporary museum has become a site and space for the articulation of social and public histories, but also for artistic expression and creation. The museum increasingly now has an educative function, and it performs this for many community and educational groups, always imagining and positioning itself within a larger world of readily available mass entertainment and information dissemination.

The medical history museum of the past had a different function. As a dedicated space for the formal education of medical students, and usually not a recognised site for public exhibitions or displays of social history, such museums often were located in or near to university medical schools, and would house a variety of specimen jars, old medical books, and material culture including medical instruments, anatomical models, body parts, skulls and images. Much of this material was collected and collated by medical administrators, doctors, academics and instructors, and the museum itself usually mirrored the work and achievements of the medical and educational institutions it represented.

To convey the challenges and opportunities presented by the medical museum for social historians of mental health, it is useful for me to outline my own experiences when I was invited to curate an exhibition about the history of mental health in the late 1990s in the traditional, static, and solid space of the medical museum, bound by its conventions of locked and glassed cabinets and display cases (Coleborne 2001). This was an exhibition at the Brownless Medical Museum at the University of Melbourne, 'A Closed World' (1998–1999). The very possibility of this exhibition in this particular space did announce a sense of change: the chance to portray psychiatric history in an exhibition—one that was given much publicity, including radio interviews, among other press coverage, and attracted sizeable visitor audiences, including regular school groups—was one to grasp. Here was a chance to convey some of the historical ideas I had about power and knowledge inside colonial mental hospitals to a wider audience, and also to bring the narrative of mental health into the twentieth century and to go beyond my original research. I chose to use patient and consumer advocacy pamphlets and images to show that the changing story of community mental health presents ongoing challenges to the dominant story of institutionalisation.

There were some difficulties created by the space of the medical museum. It was impossible for visitors to touch and interact with our sources. These were precious, on loan from Museums Victoria (MV) and drawn mostly from the Charles Brothers Collection, a significant collection of psychiatric objects named after a prominent psychiatrist in Victoria in the twentieth century.[2] Even though the MV had not expressed much willingness to display them in its own context, the items were not to be touched and handled (see Coleborne 2011, 18). The 'look but don't touch' mentality of the medical history museum environment presented barriers for some audiences. Behind glass, the records of institutionalised people were a stark, symbolic reminder of the captivity they faced in the past, and for some of the exhibition visitors, this was a negative experience. The sight of the straight-jacket, wrist cuffs, and other restraining garments generated debate among those involved in the curatorial and exhibition process. At the time, I thought it was a risk to foreground these particular material objects because of the dark past they signified: the physical restraint and control of asylum inmates (see Coleborne 2011, 25) and yet the image of me standing next to the glass case with the straight jacket inside was featured in *The Age* newspaper (30 January 1999, 41).

If we contrast this with later museum exhibitions of mental health, institutions, and histories, such as the Museum of Brisbane's exhibition *Remembering Goodna* in 2007 (Besley and Finnane 2011) or Te Awamutu Museum's *Footprints on the Land* display focused on Tokanui Hospital in the North Island of New Zealand in 2006, we can see evidence of the positive changing concept of the display of mental health history inside the space of the museum (Paisley 2009). These two exhibitions were developed and mounted at around the same time, telling us that consumer movements in mental health following institutional closures have generated shifts in our thinking about telling stories of mental illness, shifts that have had ripples that reach out and into our museums as cultural institutions.

Museums are now digital environments and have virtual presences. This change has significance for the engagement with mental health. For example, successful digital histories of mental health include online collections of mental health oral history narratives and the stunning 'suitcase' online exhibition, *The Lives They Left Behind*, which was mounted as a real exhibition in 2004 at the New York State Museum and then as a virtual museum site.[3]

Artworks help to recreate the mood and feeling of institutions, as with the Adam Art Gallery exhibition of photography, '*Still Present*'. The photographic works inspired public forums such as 'Interpreting Traces: The Construction and Representation of Psychiatric Institutions in History, Architecture and the Visual Arts', involving historians and artists in discussion about representations of madness. At the *Remembering Goodna* exhibition at the Museum of Brisbane, curated by Joanna Besley, mental health consumers were invited to create art pieces using empty first aid boxes and filling them with objects and items that resonated for them in terms of their own mental health journeys. The resulting pieces were artworks: stunning, moving, and effective as both art and as containers of memory. As historian Fiona Paisley remarked in her review of the exhibition, 'through art, painful memories can become translated into statements of resilience, humour, and hope' (Paisley 2009, 178; see also Besley and Low 2010). The therapeutic aspect of the work that went into these first aid boxes was obvious: in making something, mental health subjects had come to terms with some aspects of their own illness, care, self-care, and treatment. It was stunning: it lit up the wall.

These memories must, then, have invited powerful responses from museum visitors, who were able to contribute to these stories in an interactive collection of feedback. Visitors were also invited to respond to the *Footprints on the Land* exhibition at the Te Awamutu Museum. Its curator, Stephanie Lambert, noted that the display saw many visitors coming back several times to engage with the oral histories at listening posts and the various objects that signified much to former institutionalised people, among other aspects of the exhibition (Lambert 2012, 231–234). Evoking memories, both painful and pleasant, is, then, a critical part of any museum exhibition—but providing a means for its resolution, in the case of those suffering and visitors who require more careful signposting, is another thing altogether.[4]

These sensory, material cultures send us into a new space, writes Gaynor Kavanagh, drawing upon Sheldon Annis (Kavanagh 2000, 3). It is a dream-like space, where the senses are arrested, and where the visual power of images and objects is part of the sensory experience in the museum. This suggests new forms of interaction and belonging in museums. Visitors bring meanings and even their own objects and artworks to the museum; they certainly bring their powerful responses and feedback. This is a seismic shift that has taken place for the visitors who come with a mental health experience. Visitors with lived experiences of mental illness might also have transitioned, in many instances, from one mental health institutional site to another. In the retelling of psychiatric histories, the forbidding form and function of the museum as an institutional space is being challenged and replaced, just as the mental health institutions of the past have also been dismantled. What the future brings must be more positive for both kinds of 'institutional' structures, and for those who encounter mental health systems and treatments as consumers. Museums, then, have become sites for dissent.

Outsider art, or the art of peoples confined inside institutions or other carceral environments, provides us with other interpretive possibilities. Collections of patient artworks seem to have an ambiguous identity, especially if collected by psychiatrists as part of their work and practice over long period of time. In Melbourne, Victoria, the collection amassed by Eric Cunningham-Dax from the 1950s (see Robson 1999) is just one example of a much larger international practice among treating psychiatrists who saw therapeutic value in patient creativity. A much earlier example of patient artworks shows us that this practice has a longer history: Dr. W. A. F. Browne, the Physician Superintendent of Crichton

Royal Institution in Dumfries (1838–1857) encouraged patients to make art (McGeachan 2017, 59).

Despite its reputation and history as a prison-like institution founded on principles of control and restraint, did the asylum ever properly contain madness? Social histories of the institution for the confinement of the insane have suggested that these hospitals were carceral spaces, even while they also offered the chance for respite, safe 'asylum' from the world of distractions and harsh living, combined with moral therapies and the hope of cure for some inmates. The need for security, safety and control in the care of the insane shaped the design of institutions in most places.

Yet perhaps madness has always been *uncontained* through its very embodiment, despite the institutional physical regimes of confinement and seclusion. Late twentieth-century narratives of patient, consumer and psychiatric survivor movements provide us with the possibility of re-reading the behaviours of institutionalised peoples of the past. Former patients or inmates of institutions have been active contributors to new knowledge about these histories in public life.

These are contested histories. As Canadian historians Dyck and Deighton put it, 'scholars do not agree on how the world should remember the asylum' (Dyck and Deighton 2017, 8). Increasing opportunities to articulate the effects and impact of institutional confinement following closures have opened up the psychiatric institution to further scrutiny, and have arguably made it even more important. The legacy of the institution is profound: because of that, written accounts, visual and material traces of mental health have taken on new meanings in the 'still-present' past.

NOTES

1. See Adam Art Gallery. 2005. Still present: Exploring psychiatric institutions in photography. http://www.adamartgallery.org.nz/past-exhibitions/still-present/. Accessed 9 March 2019.
2. See Corporate Entry—Charles Brothers Museum (1950s–1980s). Encyclopedia of Australian Science. http://www.eoas.info/biogs/A002358b.htm. Accessed 9 March 2019.
3. *Lost Cases, Recovered Lives: Suitcases from a State Hospital Attic.* See Gonnerman, Jennifer. 2004. What they left behind. *The Village Voice.* https://www.villagevoice.com/2004/01/20/what-they-left-behind/.

Accessed 9 March 2019. See The Community Consortium Inc. 2015. The lives they left behind: Suitcases from a state hospital attic. http://www.suitcaseexhibit.org/index.php?section=about&subsection=exhibit. Accessed 15 March 2019.

4. See also Kenmore Hospital, Goulburn, NSW, 'The Familiars', 2004–2005. See reference to Kenmore Hospital, Goulburn NSW in Laudenbach, Cathy. 2004. The familiars: A photographic exhibition (catalogue). Canberra: Canberra Museum and Gallery.

Suggested Readings

Besley, Joanna, and Carol Low. 2010. Hurting and healing: Reflections on representing experiences of mental illness in museums. In *Re-presenting disability: Activism and agency in the museum*, eds Richard Sandell, Jocelyn Dodd, and Rosemarie Garland-Thomson, 130–142. London: Routledge.

Besley, Joanna, and Mark Finnane. 2011. Remembering Goodna: Stories from a Queensland mental hospital. In *Exhibiting madness in museums: Remembering psychiatry through collections and display*, eds Coleborne and MacKinnon, 116–136. London and New York: Routledge.

Burge, Roslyn. 2015. Callan Park in transition. In *Deinstitutionalisation and after: Post-war psychiatry in the Western world*, eds Despo Kritsotaki, Vicky Long, and Matthew Smith, 57–74. Basingstoke: Palgrave.

Coleborne, Catharine. 2001. Exhibiting "madness": Material culture and the asylum. *Health and History* 3 (2): 104–117.

Coleborne, Catharine. 2003. Remembering psychiatry's past: The psychiatric collection and its display at Porirua Hospital Museum, New Zealand. *Journal of Material Culture* 8 (1): 99–119.

Coleborne, Catharine. 2011. Collecting psychiatry's past: Collectors and their collections of psychiatric objects in Western histories. In *Exhibiting madness in museums: Remembering psychiatry through collections and display*, eds Catharine Coleborne and Dolly MacKinnon, 15–29. London and New York: Routledge.

Coleborne, Catharine. 2014. Mental health and the museum: Institutional spaces for memories and interaction. *Forum: Museums and Mental Health* 2: 162–166.

Coleborne, Catharine. 2017. An end to Bedlam? The enduring subject of madness in social and cultural history. *Social History* 42 (3): 420–429.

Coleborne, Catharine, and Dolly MacKinnon, eds. 2011. *Exhibiting madness in museums: Remembering psychiatry through collections and display*. London and New York: Routledge.

Dyck, Erika, and Alex Deighton. 2017. *Managing madness: Weyburn Mental Hospital and the transformation of psychiatric care in Canada*. Winnipeg, Canada: University of Manitoba Press.

Goffman, Erving. 1961. *Asylums: Essays on the social situation of mental patients and other inmates*. New York: Anchor Books.

Goodwin, Clare. 2004. *Shadows and silence*. Wellington, NZ: Steele Roberts.

Kavanagh, Gaynor. 2000. *Dream spaces: Memory and the museum*. London and New York: Leicester University Press.

Kritsotaki, Despo, Vicky Long, and Matthew Smith, eds. 2016. *Deinstitutionalisation and after: Post-war psychiatry in the Western world*. Basingstoke: Palgrave.

Kuglitsch, Linnea. 2018. "Kindly hearts and tender hands": Exploring the asylum and patient narratives through the archaeological record. Society for the Social History of Medicine Conference, Liverpool, UK, 11–13 July.

Lambert, Stephanie. 2012. Remembering Tokanui: Collaborative approaches to history. In *Changing times, changing places: From Tokanui hospital to mental health services in the Waikato, 1910–2012*, eds Catharine Coleborne and the Waikato Mental Health Group, 225–236. Hamilton, New Zealand: Half Court Press.

McGeachan, Cheryl. 2017. 'The Head Carver': Art extraordinary and the small spaces of asylum. *History of Psychiatry* 28 (1): 58–71.

Osborne, Ray. 2003. Asylums as cultural heritage: The challenges of adaptive re-use. In *Madness in Australia: Histories, heritage and the asylum*, eds Catharine Coleborne and Dolly MacKinnon, 217–227. St Lucia, Brisbane: University of Queensland Press.

Paisley, Fiona. 2009. Peeling back history: The remembering Goodna exhibition. Australian asylums and their histories, special issue. *Health and History* 11 (1): 172–178.

Parr, Hester, and Chris Philo. 1996. "A forbidding fortress of locks, bars and padded cells": The locational history of mental health care in Nottingham. *Historical Geography Research Series No. 32*. Edinburgh: Edinburgh University Press.

Robson, Belinda. 1999. A history of the Cunningham Dax Collection of 'psychiatric art': From art therapy to public education. *Health and History* 1 (4): 330–346.

Robson, Belinda. 2003. Preserving psychiatry through art: Historical perspectives on the Cunningham Dax Collection of psychiatric art. In *Madness in Australia: Histories, heritage and the asylum*, eds Catharine Coleborne and Dolly MacKinnon, 195–205. St Lucia: University of Queensland Press.

Sacks, Oliver. 2019 [2009]. The lost virtues of the asylum. In *Everything in its place*, 184–200. New York: Knopf; London: Picador.

Scull, Andrew. 1979. *Museums of madness: The social organization of insanity in nineteenth century England*. Middlesex: Penguin.

Scull, Andrew. 1993. *The most solitary of afflictions: Madness and society in Britain, 1700–1900*. New Haven, CT: Yale University Press.

Scull, Andrew. 1996. Asylums: Utopias and realities. In *Asylum in the community*, eds Dylan Tomlinson and John Carrier, 7–17. London and New York: Routledge.

Scull, Andrew. 2015. *Madness in civilization: A cultural history of insanity, from the bible to Freud, from the madhouse to modern medicine.* Princeton, NJ: Princeton University Press.

Taylor, Barbara. 2015 [2014]. *The last asylum: A memoir of madness in our times.* Chicago: University of Chicago Press.

Wallcraft, Jan. 1996. Some models of asylum and help in times of crisis. In *Asylum in the community*, eds Dylan Tomlinson and John Carrier, 186–206. London and New York: Routledge.

Willis, Elizabeth with Karen Twigg. 1994. *Behind closed doors: A catalogue of artefacts from Victorian psychiatric institutions held at the Museum of Victoria.* Melbourne: Museum Victoria.

Wellcome Collection. September 2016–January 2017. Bedlam: The asylum and beyond. https://wellcomecollection.org/exhibitions/W31tsSkAACkAP5p8. Accessed 31 July 2019.

Madlove: A designer asylum at Wellcome Collection's Bedlam: Asylum and beyond exhibition. 2017. http://www.madlove.org.uk/portfolio/bedlam. Accessed 31 July 2019.

CHAPTER 4

Extra-Institutional Care, or Madness Uncontained

Institutional closures created the impetus for new writing about asylums of the nineteenth and twentieth centuries, as well as other ways to represent and access these worlds and experiences for the former inmates of institutions. One of the themes that has become significant is the history of alternatives to institutional mental health care and treatment. Extra-institutional care has taken many different forms over time. This chapter turns to David Wright's question about the way that historians have often assumed the 'primacy of the mental hospital' in the past (Wright 1997, 155). In part because of their physical presence, and also because of the overwhelming amount of institutional source material for the institutions of the nineteenth century, these sites for confinement have loomed large both in public imaginations, and in the scholarship of the history of mental health. And this dominance is for good reason intellectually, too: elsewhere, I suggest that these social and medical institutions played a far greater role in narratives of place, nationhood and population than historians have really acknowledged (Coleborne 2015, 2–3).

In the face of the powerful construct of the psychiatric institution as an impermeable site, families became important points of contact for an emerging debate about the relative merits of extra-institutional care and later, deinstitutionalisation in the mid-twentieth century. The starting point for this discussion was the history of families and their uses of the asylum as an institution (Finnane 1985) and most recently, historians have been concerned to show that the asylums were more permeable than earlier studies of insanity demonstrated.

© The Author(s) 2020
C. Coleborne, *Why Talk About Madness?* Mental Health in Historical
Perspective, https://doi.org/10.1007/978-3-030-21096-0_4

Questions about how families and communities coped with insanity back inside the space of the private household, and how patients themselves may have coped with this transition, have been important interventions. In *Madness in the Family* (Coleborne 2010), I looked at the interplay between institutions and the outside world, and therefore at the *spaces between* institutionalisation. As part of that study, and in thinking about Akihito Suzuki's notion that mental breakdown was potentially threatening to families from the inside (Suzuki 2006, 121), I outlined the way that families and private households nevertheless became sites for the negotiation of the control over insanity in some instances. Nancy Tomes also argues that as families came increasingly to see institutionalisation as one solution to family domestic problems caused by the stress of mental breakdown, the asylum, too 'inevitably became the focus of familial conflicts' (Tomes 1984, 262).

Just how well the modern interpretation of care in the community has met this challenge is the subject of this chapter. Talking about other forms of care for those experiencing mental illness in this way follows a decade of historical explorations of the role of the family, its agency and negotiations with institutions. Historians show that by uncovering the extent of families' interactions with institutions, they can provide a more positive view of the asylum itself as a porous institution where families and communities moved in and out of dialogue with medical superintendents. This more positive view of the asylum has provided a rich counterpoint to the earlier more negative view of the asylum or hospital as a site of social control.

Earlier histories rendered the institutions places of control because the context for the production was the anti-psychiatry movement of the 1960s and 1970s. Yet the asylum was not the only solution to the perceived problem of mental illness in the past. Alternative possibilities for the treatment of mental illness, as well as its 'containment', can be found in people's experiences of mental breakdown in cultures where they were able to move freely and live among families, communities of friends and supporters in what some historians label as 'open care' (Mueller 2010, 172). Most famously, in the provincial Flemish town of Gheel near Antwerp, Belgium, members of the wider community cared for the mad in their homes and had done so for centuries. It was known as a 'colony for the mad', and by the end of the nineteenth century, boasted over one thousand foster families who cared for almost two thousand people (Mueller 2010, 179–181). This practice of hosting mad visitors in secular families came from the notion of the religious pilgrimage to Gheel by Saint Dymphna, the Irish saint who fled Ireland and was later named the patron saint of mental illness. Over time, this open care was regulated by guidelines such as standards of housing, and the standard of the care itself. Remuneration was offered and inspections took place. Similar models can be found in other parts of Western Europe including Italy and Norway, and also in Japan (Gijswijt-Hofstra et al. 2005, 14). Later, in the 1930s, Dutch families sent their family members to Gheel (Gijswijt-Hofstra 2005, 45). In France after 1900, separate suburbs for 'family settlements' were established allowing open and free movement for the mad who did not need to be enclosed (Coffin 2005, 226). In the more recent past, Sacks visited other residential communities in the United States, including the Gould Farm in the Berkshires, where he witnessed 'community, companionship, opportunities for work and creativity', as well as forms of medical intervention for some residents (Sacks 2019, 198–199).

The mad among the upper class were also cared for at home in England, especially in the eighteenth century. Both Akihito Suzuki and Hilary Marland write about economies of care for the wealthy who were coping with forms of madness at home (Suzuki 2006; Marland 2004). For women at home with puerperal mania, these were 'disordered households', with middle-class women becoming what Marland calls 'alarming spectres in their own homes' (Marland 2004, 65). In Asia, specifically China and Japan, different ideas about home-based care existed from the early modern era to the late 1860s, and the 'mad' were often cared for at home. Governed by rules about the sizes and spaces of confinement, such as strict dimensions of rooms as 'cells', these instances were not always exemplars of humane caring for the mad. Later, by the twentieth century, increasing urbanisation meant Japanese people moving to towns and population centres pushed the responsibility for the care and confinement of the mad onto institutions which sprang up as a response to growth in urban populations and scattered kinship and familial relations. The small institutions that were established in urban Japan tended to cater to under 100 patients, while in rural areas, family care persisted for a longer period (Suzuki 2012).

Models of family care were also investigated by asylum administrators from all over the world, including New Zealand and Australia. By the early decades of the twentieth century, these practices of trial leave, leave of absence, and probation, were regarded as very successful.

Perhaps because of the relatively high numbers of patients out on leave from institutions in each place over the course of a year, the official view on patients' leave was that it was a practice more common to the colonial world than elsewhere, and well-suited to that context. Dr. Eric Sinclair, in his Presidential Address to the Australasian Medical Congress for 1908, described the 'power to give leave of absence' as being of 'inestimable value' to convalescent patients and their families, all of whom knew they could still rely on the institution for care and assistance (Sinclair 1909, 225; Coleborne 2010, 125).

Sinclair's comments show a growing awareness of the way that mental health patients were dogged by sometimes unpredictable illness trajectories, which also formed a pattern of care. The notion that patients would still 'belong' to the asylum is also important. As historians point out, families' input into institutional care did not end with discharge, because individuals continued to be in a relationship with the institution and the wider community which had been shaped by their status as patients (Warsh 1989, 98). This is illustrated in the cases of patients reported beyond the institutional confines, sometimes when they were out on leave, supposedly enjoying the freedoms of life as recovering patients.

In the late nineteenth century, a one-time official visitor to hospitals for the insane, Mr. F. G. Ewington, gave an interview to the *New Zealand Herald*. He told the reporter that the treatment of insanity had changed to the extent that sufferers were more often released and able to resume 'normal' life. Cure was an aim of the institution. 'Frequently', he said, 'I meet people in the streets of Auckland whom I have seen in the Asylum. I always make a point of not noticing them unless they notice me first; otherwise, I might suggest painful associations' (*New Zealand Herald* 1896, 3).

Institutions were regularly petitioned by family members. Historians point out that families knew enough about these practices to want to use them, as Sinclair also noted in his 1908 address (Melling and Forsythe 2006, 113). Historians agree that families were in fact more involved with institutional care than previously imagined, and that they also demonstrated forms of agency and purpose in relation to institutional care. Not only families sought to intervene and advocate for those who were institutionalised, but also employers and friends. In the nineteenth century, forms of 'aftercare' for those patients released from hospitals provide other ways to understand community care. There were two issues at stake: both the safety of the person who had been confined, then released, and who was trying to navigate the world outside the institution; and the health of the family itself. The histories of extra-institutional care are also stories of mobility and transitions between institutions and the home.

This history of aftercare provides fresh insight into the dimensions of community and family care alongside institutions. In England, The After-care Association for Poor and Friendless Female Convalescents on Leaving Asylums for the Insane formed in 1879 as a charity.[1] In New South Wales, Australia, the Aftercare Association (1907) gave hope to many people who had been discharged from the asylums and were seeking employment, a ballast in difficult times, and surrogate familial relationships as they navigated life outside the walls of the institution (Coleborne 2010, 139–142).[2]

Shifting our attention to a later time period, this history of aftercare is a useful point of departure because it inserts a view of the worlds in between institutional confinement and familial care. Aftercare and forms of family advocacy prompt new questions about the move towards community psychiatry in the later twentieth century. Barbara Taylor's memoir links this long history to her own experience of the hostel, an in-between place of care, in the late 1980s (Taylor 2015 [2014], 189). The mid to late twentieth-century histories of community psychiatry, patient advocacy movements, anti-psychiatry and peer support, all framed by changing approaches to mental health policy, have tended to obscure the roles of families once again, placing the tussle between formal authority and informal power or different pressure groups. Yet we know that families played roles inside and outside of these groups, weaving lines between advocacy, care, intervention, fear and reliance on medical personnel for expertise, and were reliant on forms of institutional care for custody and control of sometimes unwell family members.

Examples of different architectural models of the institution can also remind us of the ways that institutions imagined spaces and places of care at least partially focused on the wellbeing of patients, as much as on 'control'. These include the villa system of the early twentieth century, popular in New Zealand, with low-slung individual buildings for groups of patients instead of large structures divided by corridors and organised into wards. Yet buildings were only part of the problem, or solution, to social change and perceptions of institutional care of those experiencing mental illness. Roy Porter offered his insights about the 'waning of the asylum era' in his broad and perceptive history of medicine

(Porter 1999, 521). Porter saw the rise of 'social psychiatry' from the late 1940s as creating a new, blurred distinction between 'sane and insane', and ushering in changes like day hospitals, regular visiting, and the 'unlocked door' policy explored by many institutions. 'Therapeutic communities', where the hierarchical nature of the institution and its practices was challenged by new practices involving patient autonomy and shared decision-making, followed (Coleborne 2003a).

Patient survivor movements sprang up around the western world from the second half of the twentieth century. Influenced by Italian psychiatrist Franco Basaglia (1924–1980) who 'opened up' institutions in Italy in the early 1960s, these movements were part of a wider anti-psychiatry discourse in the wake of some theorising by psychoanalysts including R. D. Laing and anti-colonial writer Frantz Fanon, as well as Michel Foucault and Erving Goffman (see Foot 2015). Basaglia improvised, as John Foot contends, allowing patients at the Gorizian Asylum to have a patient assembly with voting rights, and challenging the physical confines of the institution. These processes are not without their critics (notably Kathleen Jones 1993). Such radical change potentially created institutions in chaos, with families left to manage the situations of patients now 'free' from institutional care and control. In 1950s Canada, social researchers raised questions about the effects of long-term institutionalisation on people. Colleagues of Goffman at the Weyburn Mental Hospital developed concepts of the passive and imprisoned patient, concerned about the idea of populations of those suffering from mental illness who lost touch with the outside world over their 'lifetimes' inside mental hospitals (see Dyck and Deighton 2017, 149–151). As a result, Weyburn created the conditions for change: the 'dissolving of the walls' of the hospital, inspired by international examples, led to therapeutic communities like those modelled in Britain in the 1950s (Dyck and Deighton 2017, 156).

Other experimental models continued to spring up in the same period: Kingsley Hall was a therapeutic community in East London between 1965 and 1970. R. D Laing encouraged the use of this space by people experiencing schizophrenia and psychosis, and it became an infamous site of personal explorations of states of madness (see Barnes 1971). In New Zealand, at Tokanui Hospital, psychiatrist John Saxby created the Kia Tukua ward for young people which was based on similar principles of open care, patient-led therapies, and a critique of psychiatry, but in the context of a very large and diverse psychiatric institution with a population of over 1000 at that time (Coleborne 2012, 105). One person who experienced that ward described it as a 'haven': 'to come here, get some healing of some sort, clear yourself, blow the cobwebs out and go back out into the world' (Coleborne 2012, 105).

The Australian experience of community care took many forms: from government-funded services to fellowships, non-government organisations, and experimental care. While it differs across states and territories, the trajectory of community care mirrors that of other countries. The oldest Mental Health Association in Australia, The Mental Health Foundation of Australia (Victoria), was established in 1930. It is an organisation of professionals, people with lived experiences and their families, and it has links with other organisations concerned with mental health advocacy. As part of the national and international mental health movement, the Foundation signals a connection with the establishment of mental hygiene in Victoria. By the early 1950s, with English immigrant Dr. Eric Cunningham Dax taking up the role of the founding Chair of the Victorian Mental Hygiene Council (later Authority), the responses to a damning report into the experiences of institutionalised people (the Kennedy Report of 1950), was framed by a changing mindset around mental health informed by Dax's own involvement with therapeutic communities and art therapies in England.[3]

Political protest was a marked aspect of the new agency being sparked among mental health consumers around the western world. In Scotland, the Scottish Union of Mental Patients was formed following a petition of protest at conditions on the wards of Hartwood Hospital presented to Mental Welfare Commissioners in 1971 (Gallagher 2017, 102). This moment became pivotal for mental health patients across other places and showed the importance of speaking out against poor social and material conditions inside many institutions with longer histories stretching back to the nineteenth century in many instances.

In Britain, Helen Spandler suggests that there was a convergence between patient-survivor movements and other social movements of the time, especially the feminist movement (Spandler 2016). Spandler's experiences of the anti-psychiatry movement in the early 1980s were deeply personal, informed by the politics of the day (Spandler 2017). The value and importance of speaking out was widely acknowledged. In the United Kingdom, documentaries such as 'We're not mad, we're angry', first screened in 1986, later showed how important it was for mental health consumers or service users of that broad period from the

1960s and 70s of history to narrate their own experiences of the mental health system. New research projects in that vein include Diana Rose's large Wellcome Investigator grant (2016) to lead research by and for users of mental health services. 'Survivor history' groups have an important status in the narrative of mental health care and activism in the twentieth century.[4]

As the emphasis on patient autonomy increased, and many institutions closed, patient communities needed to find other forms of community and peer support. Examples of provincial consumer support and advocacy groups include the Mental Patients' Association (MPA) of Vancouver. The MPA was founded in 1971 and was the first peer support entity of its kind in Canada. The group was established primarily in response to the deinstitutionalisation process and the associated gaps in community-based care. The MPA was labelled as a radical group because its members challenged the system of psychiatry, especially the hierarchy that placed mental health consumers at the bottom. The MPA was founded as a democracy with elected positions, and participants were responsible for various initiatives such as drop-in centres, co-operative homes, research and education. By the early 1990s other groups had formed, including the mental health consumer group Mental Health Rights Coalition (MHRC) of Hamilton, Ontario (1991). Many similar groups were formed during this period, and some were eventually funded by provincial governments. The MHRC became a non-profit organisation in 1995 and continues to be governed by a volunteer Board of Directors. The Mad Pride group formed in 1993 to raise awareness of mental illness in the community and give consumers a voice. A key focus of the group's stated aims is to change the language used in relation to those with mental illness. Mad Pride is now established in seven locations across Canada and has a presence in many other countries, including Australia.[5]

In New Zealand, Mary O'Hagan was a key initiator of the psychiatric survivor movement in the late 1980s. O'Hagan describes the highly politicised nature of the peer support network and movement in New Zealand at a time when the survivor movement of the 1970s was focused on 'terrible conditions in mental hospitals and social exclusion':

> There [were] ... two arms to it: ... the advocacy and the protests, and the peer support. And a lot of very independently based peer support networks were set up and ... it was almost a bit like the feminist consciousness

raising groups; they weren't just about supporting each other – they were about blending that into an analysis of the system, the whole way people were treated. Now what's happened since then is that the system started to think: 'we need to employ people as peer support workers'. (Interview Coleborne and O'Hagan 2015)

O'Hagan goes on to describe the way that, over time, more people employed by mainstream mental health services were peer workers. However, some of those workers, she commented, lacked the critical education to understand best practice: while they focused on 'self-determination ... the importance of lived experience, knowledge, and the importance of recovery and hope', they still required appropriate mental health training to be truly effective care workers.

The post-institutional period meant that new problems became visible. Madness was now back in the public eye, where the ancient, medieval and early modern world had literally 'seen' it; whereas in the modern era, it was relatively hidden behind institutional walls. In the twentieth century, visible madness manifested through many forms of mobility including homelessness. It was compounded by issues of poverty, intersectionality, and the role of social welfare institutions such as halfway houses and shelters, and the justice system. Helen Spandler writes about the failures of 'community care' in Britain, and the lack of adequate resourcing of psychiatric interventions for those who need help: 'Despite fears of the ever increasing "psychiatrisation" of everyday life ... it is not that easy to get psychiatrised these days' (Spandler 2017). And on the efficacy of peer workers and madness in the post-institutional context, Spandler notes that 'thirty years ago we were debating post-asylum care. What would community care look like? ... Perhaps we have entered a phase of "post-community care"' (Spandler 2017).

The late modern attempts to 'contain' madness have been a commentary on the world we occupy: how do we understand and respond to mental breakdown in our midst? What can we do about it, how do we support those with severe and multiple social problems? What does it mean to speak of, or witness, madness in public? Will madness be, as Spandler suggests, 'mainstreamed' (Spandler 2017)? As we examine the socio-economic realities of madness in public places, we should also reflect on the cultural histories of seeing and hearing madness, as well as discussing the contested spaces through which we all move. The common experiences of post-institutional care across places are suggestive of a new meta-history of madness, one that examines responses to closure, but also the interventions of critics of psychiatry. Public debate about psychiatry and its past is a first step towards understanding the future possibilities for mental health care.

NOTES

1. See http://www.together-uk.org/about-us/our-history. Accessed 31 July 2019.
2. Examples of aftercare in the United States in the early twentieth century can also be found. See https://socialwelfare.library.vcu.edu/programs/mental-health/social-work-and-aftercare-of-the-mentally-ill-in-maryland/. Accessed 31 July 2019.
3. https://mhfa.org.au/CMS/OurHistory. Accessed 31 July 2019.
4. https://www.theguardian.com/society/2008/sep/03/mentalhealth. Accessed 29 July 2019.
5. http://www.torontomadpride.com/. Accessed 29 July 2019. https://nswmentalhealthcommission.com.au/events/mad-pride. Accessed 27 July 2019.

SUGGESTED READINGS

Barnes, Mary. 1971. *Mary Barnes: Two accounts of a journey through madness.* London: MacGibbon and Kee.

Coffin, Jean-Christophe. 2005. 'Misery' and 'revolution': The organisation of French psychiatry, 1900–1980. In *Psychiatric cultures compared: Psychiatry and mental health care in the twentieth century*, eds Marijke Gijswijt-Hofstra et al., 225–247. Amsterdam: Amsterdam University Press.

Coleborne, Catharine. 2003a. Preserving the institutional past and histories of psychiatry: Writing about Tokanui Hospital, New Zealand, 1950s–1990s. *Health and History* 5 (2): 104–122.

Coleborne, Catharine. 2003b. Collecting 'madness': Psychiatric collections and the museum in Victoria and Western Australia. In *Madness in Australia: Histories, heritage and the asylum*, eds Catharine Coleborne and Dolly MacKinnon, 183–194. St Lucia: University of Queensland Press.

Coleborne, Catharine. 2010. *Madness in the family: Insanity and institutions in the Australasian colonial world, 1860–1914.* Basingstoke and New York: Palgrave Macmillan.

Coleborne, Catharine. 2012. Patient journeys: Stories of mental health care from Tokanui to mental health services, 1930s to the 1980s. In *Changing times, changing places: From Tokanui to mental health services in the Waikato, 1910–2012*, ed. Catharine Coleborne, 97–103. Hamilton: Half Court Press.

Coleborne, Catharine. 2015. *Insanity, identity and empire: Colonial institutional confinement in Australia and New Zealand, 1870–1910*. Manchester: Manchester University Press.

Dyck, Erika, and Alex Deighton. 2017. *Managing madness: Weyburn mental hospital and the transformation of psychiatric care in Canada*. Winnipeg, Canada: University of Manitoba Press.

Finnane, Mark. 1985. Asylums, families and the state. *History Workshop Journal* 20 (1): 134–148.

Foot, John. 2015. *The man who closed the asylums: Franco Basaglia and the revolution in mental health care*. London: Verso.

Gallagher, Mark. 2017. From asylum to action in Scotland: The emergence of the Scottish Union of Mental Patients, 1971–2. *History of Psychiatry* 28 (1): 101–114.

Gijswijt-Hofstra, Marijke. 2005. Within and outside the walls of the asylum: Caring for the Dutch mentally ill, 1884–2000. In *Psychiatric cultures compared: Psychiatry and mental health care in the twentieth century*, eds Marijke Gijswijt-Hofstra et al., 35–72. Amsterdam: Amsterdam University Press.

Gijswijt-Hofstra, Marijke, Harry Oosterhuis, Joost Vijselaar, and Hugh Freeman. 2005. *Psychiatric cultures compared: Psychiatry and mental health care in the twentieth century*. Amsterdam: Amsterdam University Press.

Jones, Kathleen. 1993. *Asylums and after: A revised history of the mental health services: From the early 18th century to the 1990s*. London and New Brunswick, NJ: Athlone Press.

Marland, Hilary. 2004. *Dangerous motherhood: Insanity and childbirth in Victorian Britain*. Basingstoke and New York: Palgrave.

Melling, Jo, and Bill Forsythe. 2006. *The politics of madness: The state, insanity and society in England, 1845–1914*. London and New York: Routledge.

Mueller, Thomas. 2010. Re-opening a closed file of the history of psychiatry: Open care and its historiography in Belgium, France and Germany, c. 1880–1980. In *Transnational psychiatries: Social and cultural histories of psychiatry in comparative perspective c. 1800–2000*, eds Waltraud Ernst and Thomas Mueller, 172–199. Newcastle Upon Tyne: Cambridge Scholars Publishing.

O'Hagan, Mary. 2014. *Madness made me: A memoir*. Wellington, New Zealand: Open Box.

O'Hagan, Mary. 2017. Madness in New Zealand: A conversation. *Asylum: The Magazine for Democratic Psychiatry* 24 (2): 12–13.

Porter, Roy. 1999. *The greatest benefit to mankind: A medical history of humanity from antiquity to the present*. London: Fontana Press/HarperCollins.

Rose, Diana. 2017. Service user/survivor-led research in mental health: Epistemological possibilities. *Disability and Society* 32 (6): 773–789.

Sacks, Oliver. 2019 [2009]. The lost virtues of the asylum. In *Everything in its place*, 184–200. New York: Knopf; London: Picador.

Sinclair, Eric. 1909. Presidential address. *Transactions of the Australasian Medical Congress*. Melbourne, Government Printer: 225.

Spandler, Helen. 2016. Asylum magazine: 30 years of speaking out and what's changed? Voices of Madness Conference, University of Huddersfield, UK, 15–16 September.

Spandler, Helen. 2017. From psychiatric abuse to psychiatric neglect? *Asylum Magazine* 23.2. https://asylummagazine.org/2017/09/from-psychiatric-abuse-to-psychiatric-neglect-by-helen-spandler-2/. Accessed July 2019.

Suzuki, Akihito. 2006. *Madness at home: The psychiatrist, the patient, and the family in England 1820–1860*. Berkeley: University of California Press.

Suzuki, Akihito. 2012. Between two psychiatric regimes: Migration and psychiatry in early twentieth-century Japan. In *Migration, ethnicity, and mental health: International perspectives, 1840–2010*, eds Angela McCarthy and Catharine Coleborne, 141–156. London: Routledge.

Taylor, Barbara. 2015 [2014]. *The last asylum: A memoir of madness in our times*. Chicago: University of Chicago Press.

Tomes, Nancy. 1984. *A generous confidence: Thomas Story Kirkbride and the art of asylum-keeping, 1840–1883*. Cambridge: Cambridge University Press.

Warsh, Cheryl Krasnick. 1989. *Moments of unreason: The practice of Canadian psychiatry and the Homewood Retreat, 1883–1923*. Montreal and Kingston, Canada: McGill-Queen's University Press.

Wright, David. 1997. Getting out of the asylum: Understanding the confinement of the insane in the nineteenth century. *Social History of Medicine* 10 (1): 137–155.

Special interviews. Treatment of the insane: Chat with an official visitor. 1896. *New Zealand Herald*, May 20. https://paperspast.natlib.govt.nz/newspapers/NZH18960520.2.6. Accessed 1 August 2019.

Documentaries

Eleventh Hour. 1986. We're Not Mad We're Angry. Posted 31 July 2012. https://www.youtube.com/watch?v=qD36m1mveoY. Accessed July 2019.

CHAPTER 5

Talking About Mental Health and the Politics of Madness

So far, this book has suggested that talking about madness is possible through the archives of institutions, personal stories, the spaces and places of confinement and living histories of these, through exhibition, artworks and through advocacy and community support. In all of this, the politics of talking about madness has been implicit. This chapter makes a specific case for the explicit telling of historical stories in public and political spaces: for instance, through formal official commissions of inquiry into mental health institutions in the recent past. Where the new mad studies explore the idea of public education around mental health, it has promoted 'historical memory work' to liberate readers and thinkers from present constructions of mental health (LeFrançois, Menzies and Reaume 2013, 15).

The chapter takes as its feature example the Confidential Forum for Former In-Patients of Psychiatric Hospitals in New Zealand (2004–2006) and situates this within a larger global context for 'truth-telling' about institutional confinement. This Forum was followed in late 2018 by the New Zealand Government Inquiry into Mental Health and Addiction, the outcomes of which are also described here.[1] Elsewhere I have argued that the individual and collective journeys into mental health care and out the other side again have changed dramatically over the past century of mental health provision (Coleborne 2012, 97–98). The very identity of the 'patient' has changed over time, with a shift from the nineteenth-century understanding of the asylum 'inmate', with its custodial implications, to a twentieth-century reinterpretation of the

© The Author(s) 2020
C. Coleborne, *Why Talk About Madness?* Mental Health in Historical
Perspective, https://doi.org/10.1007/978-3-030-21096-0_5

'consumer' of mental health services, a term reflecting the nature of mental health care beyond institutional confines.

These various shifts in nomenclature also reflect changing patterns of legislation around committal and hospitalisation. Most users of mental health services are now outpatients, and only a small group of seriously ill people is kept inside an institutional setting, either in forensic institutional contexts or for short stays inside smaller hospital wards dedicated to psychiatric care. In the present context of mental health care, navigating the tensions between 'official' or biomedical accounts, and service user or consumer histories of mental health, results in an interesting and new politics of knowledge for the academic historian.

In the wake of deinstitutionalisation and institutional closures in most western countries, a variety of opportunities for the discussion of mental health care in the past have emerged through both formal and informal opportunities for the critique of state-run psychiatric facilities. Different narratives of mental health care have been created in these spaces: through patient advocacy and rights groups (Davies et al. 2016); through the collation of published materials (Dunst 2016); through documentaries about psychiatric institutions, and through formal inquiries. All of this points to the emergence of a powerful collective 'voice' and social movement, as Chapter 4 introduced; what scholars have analysed as speech made possible by the formation of a collective identity or habitus for consumers of mental health treatment services (Crossley and Crossley 2001, 1478).

Internationally, processes similar to the Confidential Forum in New Zealand created a space for the articulation of counter-narratives to the official story of institutionalisation. This involved some pain in the retelling for narrators. It is vital to understand that the politics of past institutions linger in the present: the long shadow of the institutions, both figurative and literal, means that mental illness is often mostly understood through the institutions which attempted to contain it. Various case studies of mental health jurisdictions remind us that the public nature of inquiries and reports sometimes also led to increased dissent, surveillance of the mentally ill in the community, and therefore heightened sense of the stigmatisation of mental illness, rather than the more hopeful outcome of improved status for people with mental illness. However, media reports about the state of mental health, and the fate of patients in the mental health care systems, remind us of the value of an open approach to the telling of stories about mental health from all sides. The range of national characterisations of mental health policy and awareness also created new social movements and champions of mental health advocacy.

Surveying the transnational field across places including the United Kingdom, the Republic of Ireland, Canada, the United States, Australia and New Zealand tells us that many transformations in understandings of mental health took place from the 1950s in western nations (Kritsotaki 2016, 6–7; 23; 27). These involved revisiting mental health legislation, rethinking policies as concepts of institutional care were changing, and new ideas about practices of care and aftercare. Formal inquiries and the reactions to these provide an important source of historical data, rich for analysis. It is in evidence provided to such inquiries that historians can locate new voices of dissent and recovery, memory and loss in the experience of psychiatric treatment.

What's the status of the different voices? Do narratives collated through formal inquiries have more credence than others? What about memoir, accounts of mental suffering and institutional violence as experienced by individuals? How can we understand these many layers of epistemology or 'knowing' about institutions and about mental illness? Oral histories provide another important avenue of inquiry. These stories allow us insights into the different worlds of the confined. Such stories provide powerful, insider perspectives of personal histories often told from outside, most often from the point of view of psychiatrists themselves. In the United Kingdom, Kerry Davies (2001) interviewed 21 patients in the public mental health system in Oxfordshire. The resulting study of their narratives is a rich piece of analysis of mental health testimonies obtained through oral histories, still rare in this field of study. As Davies notes, 'the history of psychiatry is one of the multiple narratives—professional and cultural, legal and social, those of patients and those of psychiatrists' (Davies 2001, 267).

Crossley writes about 'researching resistance' that grew up around psychiatry and mental health services in Britain in the second half of the twentieth century as a result of contention of the meanings of institutional closures (2006). Crossley suggests that the 'field of contention' was constituted by 'the interactions of competing and conflicting agents who sought to transform both conceptions and practices within the mental health system and the treatment of the "mentally ill" within wider society' (2006, 1). He argues that much of this must be understood within the neoliberal context for health care and the recasting of mental health patients precisely as 'consumers' (2006, 62). Historian Geoffrey Reaume, mentioned earlier in this book, prefers the label of 'mad'. Significantly, Crossley understands that there were networks of survivors and international connections among mental health consumers, so that these were isolated events but global in scope. Likewise, in her book, *Talking Back to Psychiatry*, Linda J. Morrison writes about the consumer/survivor/ex-patient movement, providing a useful historical background (2005, 57). Morrison stresses the role of advocacy, access to information, and the role of the activist. Morrison also situates types of psychiatric narratives, a topic that some scholarly work in New Zealand has addressed (see Campion 2009).

New Zealand's history of mental health provides us with a specific case study. As mental health advocate Mary O'Hagan explained in her interview with me in 2015, New Zealand was both like other nations, and yet also very different when it came to deinstitutionalisation:

Cathy: In your memoir, … there's a chapter on global madness. And you put New Zealand into a much bigger picture in that story. I'm just wondering if you could reflect on New Zealand within that larger context?
Mary: Going to mental health systems around the world … around the richer countries, they're all much the same … there's the same model. I remember going to a mental hospital in Britain and saying 'well it's all the same except the plugs'. You know, the electrical sockets. But what New Zealand did that no other whole country has done is that it closed down the big asylums. It didn't just downsize them, it closed them. Although there are a few exceptions there … and the next thing that New Zealand did after a few crises with a few guys getting out with guns and scaring the community was, and after the second Mason Review, they put a lot of money out into community health. (Interview Coleborne and O'Hagan 2015)

New Zealand's deinstitutionalisation era, which saw most institutions facing closure from the 1980s, brought changes for people whose experiences of the 'community' and community care would be drastically different. The most important shift in this wider debate about deinstitutionalisation occurred in the 1970s, when the Health department as a whole took what some describe as a more 'community-oriented turn' in its official reports. The trend was towards a lessening reliance on hospitalisation for those experiencing mental illness.

At different New Zealand institutions, the practice of liaising with the community and breaking down the barriers between community and institution had begun the process of eventual institutional closures in the 1980s, which was completed by the 1990s, though some institutions remained partially functional at that time. There were turning points in New Zealand's process of deinstitutionalisation. Institutional closures came in the wake of the 'Committee of Inquiry into Procedures used in Certain Psychiatric Hospitals in Relation to Admission, Discharge or Release on Leave of Certain Classes of Patient' and its Mason Report, as it became known, of 1988. The Mason Report was named after its Chairman Kenneth Mason, a District Court Judge. It detailed the serious concerns held by the public and government about crimes, including homicide, committed by mentally ill persons while outside institutions on periods of leave, as well as long-standing criticisms of treatment practices inside psychiatric facilities. Some high-profile cases were given much attention in the background explanation to the Inquiry and its subsequent report.

The implications of the Mason Report would be felt by all psychiatric institutions in the lead-up to the deinstitutionalisation of many patients in New Zealand by the late 1990s. What became very clear in the multiple recommendations of the report was that a distinction needed to be drawn between forensic in-patients and other recipients of psychiatric care. Given that processes to enable out-patient community care already existed, there was some emphasis also on the community care provided to those on leave and released from psychiatric facilities. Māori patients were also singled out as a specific social group of the mentally ill requiring additional levels of support in community care and in forensic psychiatric care.

The public nature of the Inquiry and the Mason Report led to increased debate, surveillance of the mentally ill in the community, and therefore an increased degree of the public stigmatisation of mental illness. The wider social and cultural context for the Forum is also instructive. At the time of the imminent closure of the North Island institution of Tokanui in the Waikato in 1997, a television documentary featured members of an activist group formed to fight the closure, showing how different feelings about the place ran high, and was broadcast as 'Asylum or Sanctuary?' as an episode of the current affairs programme 'Frontline' on TVNZ in May 1994. Media reports about the state of mental health, and the fate of those people in the mental health care system in New Zealand, pointed to the value of an open approach to the telling of stories about mental health from all sides.

In the 2000s, several newspaper articles about another institution in the North Island, Porirua Hospital (1887–2007) near the capital city of Wellington raised awareness about mental health treatments and poor hospital conditions. Leading up to the Confidential Forum in 2004, former staff and patients of several mental health facilities spoke about the fear created inside such institutions through treatments including electro-convulsive therapy (ECT). By 2006, in the wake of historical knowledge about Tokanui created through a museum exhibition and the oral narratives project, Tokanui, too, became the subject of discussion in the local media. In the *Waikato Times*, former staff and patients were once again interviewed about their experience of the psychiatric institution which was finally closed in 1998.

Given this history, the example of New Zealand's Confidential Forum for Former In-Patients of Psychiatric Hospitals provides a highly useful illustration of the missed potential for talking in more detail about mental health in public life at that particular point in time. In the mid-2000s, New Zealand's Labour government, under the leadership of Prime Minister Helen Clark, held mobile hearings in the major towns and cities of the two islands of the country. Known as The Confidential Forum, it was announced by the New Zealand government in 2004 and established in 2005. Its purpose was to provide a space for former in-patients, who spent time in the nation's mental health institutions prior to 1992, to speak confidentially about their experiences to a sympathetic forum. Some family members were also given the opportunity to speak. A small panel of experts with experience of the mental health system listened to evidence given by 493 people. This process took place over a period of 154 days and in more than 20 different locations around New Zealand between 2005 and 2007. Most of those who came forward to speak were former in-patients, with around 17 per cent of hearings involving the family members of former in-patients, and a small number of staff also spoke to the Forum.

This Forum was not an inquiry, but rather an attempt at reconciliation for former in-patients and families, especially those whose experiences of the mental health institutions were negative and required some follow-up treatment such as counselling referrals or, in some cases, access to legal advice. The formal outcome of this Forum, *Te Āiotanga*, was a 64-page report published in June 2007. While some members of the psychiatric community still harbour criticisms of this process, the Forum was a first for New Zealand and potentially represented a significant positive step for former in-patients of institutions.

Te Āiotanga contained digested testimony, feedback about the process, follow up actions, and appendices of information about institutional care. However, mental health advocates continue to claim that this report was never 'acknowledged' by the government, despite the fact that it was welcomed by the then Deputy Prime Minister Michael Cullen and the Health Minister Pete Hodgson in June of 2007. Some anecdotal reactions from the mental health community suggest that this might be because one reason for the Forum was that over 200 court cases had been instigated by formerly institutionalised people claiming forms of abuse, and seeking substantial compensation payments. The sense that the Forum offered only symbolic redress lingered in the background.

Being able to talk and tell stories of mental health has been established by professionals as one route to recovery, well-being and reconciliation. The Confidential Forum opened up the possibility to a variety of people for 'talk'. Almost twenty pages of the report were devoted to a summary of patients' accounts of their experiences under thematic headings including institutional culture (admission, physical conditions, routines, communication, care and compassion, consent, violence, sexual misconduct, discharge practices); treatment regimes (seclusion, ECT, medication); experiences of particular groups (children and adolescents; mothers; those with intellectual disability; transgender); and impact of experiences (summarised as shame, loss of dignity, flashbacks, grief, stigmatisation, low self-esteem, lack of stability and poor relationships).

The Confidential Forum did not make these narratives available in full following their airing during the Forum. Instead, one other outcome was the establishment of a 'Confidential listening and assistance service' which was open to anyone who wanted to talk about their experiences of different forms of state care before 1992. The connections between the longer histories of stories of abuse and ill-treatment of children in state care meant that the scope of the 'listening' was made even broader. In addition, a new emphasis was placed on patients' rights advocacy beyond the Forum itself.

There was only one member of the Forum's panel who was herself a consumer of mental health services. Anne Helm came away from the process of the Forum profoundly disillusioned by the lack of a formal apology, and with others, continues to advocate for an apology as a way forward following the Forum hearings. Participants sometimes found the process harrowing, with one woman claiming that telling her story was tantamount to reliving experiences of abuse (Helm 2014). International comparisons were also drawn, for instance to the Commission to Inquire into Child Abuse (Ireland 2000–2009).

By 2010, after the Forum took place, new debates about the safety of the community emerged following local events in Hamilton in New Zealand's central North Island involving a psychiatric out-patient. This time, a variety of views were canvassed which aimed to shed new light on the purpose and function of 'community care' of the mentally ill. Similarly, the Ministry of Health's Mental Health Foundation organisation, 'Like Minds, Like Mine', established in 1997, began to produce online and print materials devoted to reducing stigma for people with mental illness by profiling the stories of those living with mental health conditions.

Examining such episodes, events and official interventions into mental health and their surrounding referential contexts demonstrates the purpose, meaning and relevance of 'the patient narrative', and how it can contribute to the international historical documentation of mental health. Although in New Zealand in the mid-2000s the words and voices of people with mental illness were obscured by their confidential status at the Forum, since that time, by the Government Inquiry into Mental Health and Addiction in 2018, there has been an enormous shift in the thinking about the value of the 'voices of the people' as cited in the Inquiry's report, *He Ara Oranga* (2018). Whereas the earlier failure to include the published narratives of those who spoke to the Confidential Forum stood in stark contrast to other formal inquiries in different jurisdictions, including Australia, in *He Ara Oranga*, the Inquiry panel members drew on the advice of Judge Mason, who recommended listening to the people, more than twenty years after his reports of 1995–1996.

One comparison can be drawn between the Forum and the work to address the histories of Aboriginal child removal in Australia in the mid to late 1990s. The *Bringing Them Home* Report (1997) included the rich oral testimonies of people affected by long periods of colonial, state and federal policies of child removal and welfare approaches to the historical 'assimiliation' of Indigenous Australians. This report became a lightning rod for cultural redress at all levels, with profound impacts on national cultures of understanding the experiences of the nation's First Peoples.[2] In the same way, *He Ara Oranga* is a long and detailed report in 214 pages that captures the words of many of the 2000 people and over 5000 submissions made during the 2018 Inquiry. The firsthand narratives of mental illness and personal struggles are represented in the report, making it a powerful tool for change:

> We heard from tāngata whaiora; literally, people seeking wellness. They talked about their struggle to access help for mental distress and addictions and evoked the image of being 'up to their necks in deep water'. People shared deeply personal experiences, motivated by a desire to tell their stories and bring about change. (*He Ara Oranga* 2018, 35)

The result of this report, with its stories and account of madness put at the centre of the discussion, is a far deeper appreciation of the problem and also its potential solutions for all New Zealanders, with the 2019 budget promising to address the Inquiry's major recommendation for a national Mental Health and Wellbeing Commission.[3]

To bring the New Zealand case into a wider perspective, these forms of 'talk' and conversation are happening around the world. In Canada, collections of psychiatric survivor narratives have patterned the mad movement. Books such as *Shrink Resistant* (1988), *Upstairs in the Crazy House* (1992) and *Call me Crazy* (1997), like the many examples from New Zealand and other countries mentioned in this book, go some way to fleshing out the relevance of this concept of the political power of talk and opening up about madness as an experience. In England, the writer and mental health campaigner Jonny Benjamin is among many others who have committed their memories to forms of writing and communication for the public to better understand the healing possibilities of words (Benjamin 2012).

How should we listen to, and hear, these stories? Future public research and engagement through scholarship needs to consider the influence of digital technology and how this has coincided with the closures of institutions, and also helped to facilitate the idea of 'voices' and new stories of mental illness. Now that individuals have greater access, larger audiences and opportunities to share their narratives, is the stigma around mental illness also dissolving? In the twenty-first century, accessible digital narratives might help to break down barriers, just as physical barriers were removed with the opening up and closure of hospitals in the twentieth century.

Notes

1. https://www.mentalhealth.inquiry.govt.nz/. Accessed 9 August 2019.
2. See https://www.humanrights.gov.au/our-work/bringing-them-home-report-1997. Accessed 2 August 2019.
3. https://www.health.govt.nz/our-work/mental-health-and-addictions/government-inquiry-mental-health-and-addiction. Accessed 9 August 2019.

Suggested Readings

Benjamin, J. 2012. *Pill after Pill.* London: Chipmunka Publishing.
Brennan, Nicola. 2010. Playing mind games. *Waikato Times*, March 27.
Burstow, Bonnie, and Don Weitz eds. 1988. *Shrink resistant: The struggle against psychiatry in Canada.* Vancouver: New Star Books.
Campion, Michelle. 2009. "Articulate others": The significance of patient pathography in New Zealand mental health history, 1950–2008. Unpublished Masters thesis in History, University of Waikato.
Capponi, Pat. 1992. *Upstairs in the crazy house: The life of a psychiatric survivor.* Toronto: Viking Press.
Coleborne, Catharine. 2003. Preserving the institutional past and histories of psychiatry: Writing about Tokanui Hospital, New Zealand, 1950s–1990s. *Health & History* 5 (2): 104–122.
Coleborne, Catharine. 2004. "Like a family where you fight and you roar": Inside the 'personal and social' worlds of Tokanui Hospital, New Zealand, through an oral history project. *Oral History in New Zealand* 16: 17–27.
Coleborne, Catharine. 2012. Patient Journeys: Stories of mental health care from Tokanui to mental health services, 1930s to the 1980s. In *Changing times, changing places: From Tokanui to mental health services in the Waikato, 1910–2012*, ed. Catharine Coleborne, 97–109. Hamilton: Half Court Press.
Crossley, Michele, and Nick Crossley. 2001. 'Patient' voices, social movements and the habitus: How psychiatric survivors 'speak out'. *Social Science and Medicine* 52 (2001): 1477–1489.
Crossley, Nicholas. 2006. *Contesting psychiatry: Social movements in mental health.* Oxfordshire, UK and New York, NY: Routledge.
Davies, Kerry. 2001. "Silent and censured travellers"? Patients' narratives and patients' voices: Perspectives on the history of mental illness since 1948. *Social History of Medicine* 14 (2): 267–292.
Davies, Megan et al. 2016. After the asylum in Canada: Surviving deinstitutionalisation and revising history. In *Deinstitutionalisation and after: Post-war psychiatry in the Western world*, eds Despo Kritsotaki, Vicky Long, and Matthew Smith, 75–95. Basingstoke: Palgrave.

Department of Internal Affairs. *Te Āiotanga: Report of the confidential forum for former in-patients of psychiatric hospitals*. Wellington, New Zealand, June 2007.

Dunst, Alexander. 2016. All the fits that's news to print: Deinstitutionalisation and anti-psychiatric movement magazines in the United States, 1970–1986. In *Deinstitutionalisation and after: Post-war psychiatry in the Western world*, eds Despo Kritsotaki, Vicky Long, and Matthew Smith, 57–74. Basingstoke: Palgrave.

He Ara Oranga: Report of the Government Inquiry into Mental Health and Addiction. 2018. https://mentalhealth.inquiry.govt.nz/inquiry-report/he-ara-oranga/.

Helm, Anne. 2014. Te Āiotanga: A place of healing: Advancing the call for official recognition of historic abuse in Psychiatric 'care'. Human Rights Commission Roundtable: Titiri Whakamuri; Haere Whakamuru ('Look backwards, and go forward. Look to the past to build your action, and planning for the future'.)

Kritsotaki et al. 2016. *Deinstitutionalisation and after: Post-war psychiatry in the Western world*. Basingstoke: Palgrave.

LeFrançois, Brenda A., Robert Menzies, and Geoffrey Reaume, eds. 2013. *Mad matters: A critical reader in Canadian mad studies*. Toronto: Canadian Scholars' Press.

MacKinnon, Dolly, and Catharine Coleborne, eds. 2003. Deinstitutionalisation Special Issue. *Health and History* 5 (2): 1–16.

Mason, K., H. Bennett, and E. Ryan. 1988. Report of the committee of inquiry into procedures used in certain psychiatric hospitals in relation to admission, discharge or release on leave of certain classes of patients (psychiatric report). Wellington, New Zealand: Ministry of Health.

Morrison, Linda J. 2005. *Talking back to psychiatry: The psychiatric consumer/survivor/ex-patient movement*. New York: Routledge.

Shimrat, Irit. 1997. *Call me crazy: Stories from the mad movement*. Vancouver: Press Gang.

Taylor, Phil. 2004. Patients lived in fear of 'The Treatment'. *Weekend Herald*, July 10. https://www.nzherald.co.nz/nz/news/article.cfm?c_id=1&objectid=3577616. Accessed 1 August 2019.

Thorley, Lester. 2006. Return to Tokanui. *Waikato Times*, July 8.

Welch, Denis. 2003. In two minds. *The Listener*, December 13.

Resource Examples

Like minds, like mine. 2019. http://www.likeminds.org.nz. Accessed 3 March 2019.

Mental Health Foundation of New Zealand. 2019. www.mentalhealth.org.nz. Accessed 3 March 2019.

CHAPTER 6

What's the Story?

Vast numbers of people were institutionalised around the world over the nineteenth and twentieth centuries; their lives have enormous significance to local, national and global histories. The pattern for social historians to locate, sample and analyse large amounts of patient clinical case data from former institutions—the 'lives in the asylum record'—has been a well-established research mode from the 1960s, one that derived in part from institutional closures as well as from social-historical practices of the twentieth century (McCarthy et al. 2017, 360–362). Historians have managed to retrieve aspects of the patients' experience from such clinical data, although it is circumscribed and shaped by confinement and lack of freedom. The opportunity to see, hear and understand confined inmates' points of view has not been entirely impossible; cases provide some sense of language, images and notes about the insane, as well as their own words. Archival collections such as these often contain patient and family letters which are a substantial source of additional information and allow historians to look again at the insane from different angles; how the mad interacted with doctors, their families, and how the relationships between these different individuals and groups functioned. Archival collections are increasingly being digitised and made more accessible to researchers, families and interested members of the public. In 2014, the Wellcome Trust announced the enormous digitisation partnership project with a series of English and Scottish archives to digitise mental health records of the nineteenth and twentieth century, a time period that also allows for the demonstration

© The Author(s) 2020

C. Coleborne, *Why Talk About Madness?* Mental Health in Historical Perspective, https://doi.org/10.1007/978-3-030-21096-0_6

of change over time from institutional to other forms of mental health care.[1] The process is still incomplete, but promises to be a significant boost to researchers' access to these records over time.[2]

The dominance of the 'asylum' in histories of madness has situated our historical understandings of mental illness inside a model that has both acknowledged the power relations embedded in mental health treatments of the past, and yet also presents complex interpretative issues for the present. Madness is no longer contained, if it ever was, by institutional norms and practices, nor by its specific spaces for confinement. Historians of madness in England, America and Europe have argued that patients' own writings about their experiences of confinement can be construed as narratives of resistance to the asylum and its treatments of their 'madness', suggesting that 'medical historians could profit by an examination of women's diaries and letters' in their histories of psychological distress (Tomes 1990, 171; see also Rothman 1994, 1–2; 9).

In my interview with New Zealand mental health advocate Mary O'Hagan in 2015, I asked her why she thought it was important to tell the stories of mental illness in public. She replied:

> People often say about history in the bigger context that it's the narrative of the victors, the people who triumphed, who won, in whatever way or means. And I think mental health history's just the same; it's the narrative of the powerful and you don't get a well-rounded picture. And ... the narrative of the powerful will be very forgiving about the harms and the mistakes they make ... and quite often in total denial. (Interview Coleborne and O'Hagan 2015)

O'Hagan was alluding here to her knowledge of the practice of social history and its work to tell the stories of history 'from below'. She also points to her own struggle with the mental health system, a system that continually reaffirmed and told the story of experience *for* those who have experienced mental illness rather than seeking them out to tell their own side of the story of institutional care. To some extent, some readers might consider the social history practice of finding archival traces and retrieving the 'voices' of patients, and writing *about* asylums and patients, very much still stuck in an older paradigm of knowledge-making about the history of madness from the viewpoints of the powerful. As I have suggested in this book, challenges to my own work as a historian of madness and institutions have rightly (and gently) come from people with lived experiences of mental illness; especially from people who have spent time in institutions themselves. This is because their reaction to scholarly attempts at retrieval, visibility and recognition of the patient identity is that it can come across as patronising or as an appropriation of knowledge. For them, archival histories fail to fully realise a new way of seeing and understanding the history of madness from the insider's perspective.

Yet, as this book has also described, historians and other writers do see and argue that the act of investigating archival records in the service of the 'patient's view' might also perform a liberation of the captive narratives of past institutional experiences. My aim here has been to look at and engage the multiple registers of storytelling available to our new histories of madness—from the archives to the material world, to the lived experiences and protests of advocates and peer support workers—and back towards policymakers and change agents in the mental health system. When we consider that in the past, patients' utterances, writings and depositions were considered to be 'irredeemable babble' (see Porter 2002, 156), the power of the act of retrieval is more obvious and can be positioned historically. Letters to and from institutions were censored; mail from patients to the outside world was not always sent; and the rare moments and opportunities to 'hear' patients speak are often in a context of formal inquiry or under duress. One patient in the nineteenth-century asylum in colonial Australia, Maria Murray, told the Board of the formal inquiry into the Kew Metropolitan Asylum (Victoria) in 1876 that she enjoyed singing, aware that it had become definitive of her madness: 'I have been singing sometimes, not in a naughty way, but just practising for myself', she told the Board. Brought by the police to Kew Asylum, singing, Murray was told she was 'out of [her] mind'; 'but I was not out of mind', she said.[3]

In the same year that I interviewed O'Hagan, in April 2015, a story about the documentary 'Alison's Story: 50 years Under the System' appeared in the *New Zealand Herald*. It reminds us of the power of stories to create change. 'It is the raw, courageous and sensitive account of the past', writes Qiujing Wong, 'that offers us a window of hope into social change for the future' (Wong 2015). The film Mental Notes (2012), by New Zealand filmmaker Jim Marbrook, had already stimulated a service-users' perspective on the story of mental health institutions in New Zealand, with the dominant narrative shaped by survivors of the experiences of confinement, the terror and pain of what some people endured inside, and the dark humour made possible as they reflected on the past of institutions in their own words, and on their own terms.

Reflecting on the history of psychiatry, Roy Porter wrote that it is far more complex than any one viewpoint can convey: neither a 'benign vision of progress' nor a 'callous exploitation and social control' (Porter 2004, 204). In light of this complexity, this book has aimed to showcase storytelling about mental health in different genres—including academic writing—for change and social justice. In 2015, Judi Clements of the Mental Health Care Foundation of New Zealand wrote that journalism about mental health patients in facilities is lacking in nuance and balance (Clements 2015). This book has set out to generate new ideas to help with that perception; it does so by unlocking the range of histories that might be told in the present era in public settings. If we accept the view that the history of psychiatry is one of multiple narratives (Davies 2001, 267) then we need to account for the multiplicity of authors and story-tellers in this field.

The different modes of writing about the history of madness through archival traces, published narratives, and material culture, represented here point to the potential for new research strategies to better represent the problem of madness in the past and present. In this way, the book engages with the question of the possibility of a longer tradition of resistance to psy-interventions and discourses (see Coleborne in Kilty and Dej eds 2018). The reclamation of names, words and identities—the very language of psychiatry—has been instrumental to this shift.

My research for this book has uncovered at least 20 conferences, symposia and workshops reflecting on 'mad studies' held between 2014 and 2019 (see Appendix A). From Scotland, England, Ireland and the United States to Europe, Canada, Australia and New Zealand, this new emergent field of inquiry which engages communities of practice and those with lived experiences of mental illness has the power to reshape the intellectual terrain. At the 'Voices of Madness' conference held at the University of Huddersfield in 2016, I commented on my early experience as a doctoral student delivering a paper in 1996, where conference delegates had suggested to me that the study of asylums and insanity was already 'over'.[4] Not only were they incorrect, they were unable to see the links between this field and what it was to go on to become or provoke in a much wider historical domain, as I have been showing here. Significantly, these conferences, workshops, symposia and other events lean on the word 'madness', evoke critical disability studies as a field, and also signal interdisciplinary approaches and solutions to the question of mental health and its histories. There is a useful repurposing of language and words such as 'crazy', and organisers have sought to 'make sense' of and mediate madness, as well as engaging activist narratives, and also stories of resistance, suggesting new shaping forces and collaborations between communities and the world of academic inquiry.

These intellectual sites for discovery have also opened up new ways of telling stories including film, poetry and performance, moving away from the problematic construction of the asylum and 'patient', and towards a lived-experience narrative of madness. These events also suggest alternative ways of knowing, understanding and rendering historicity for madness, and point to the experience of colonisation, marginalisation and contestation, the very politics of madness described in this book.

The debates and conversations about madness and its history and present also take place online through blogs, podcasts, webinars, Facebook groups, Twitter handles, and on YouTube (see Appendix B). The democracy of digital communication has afforded groups, communities and networks different strategies for outreach and connectivity. Examples include the use of open-source digital application formats for storytelling, video and audio resources, websites, blogs and groups, such as Wordpress, Blogspot, YouTube and Facebook. *Asylum Magazine*, with its long history of engaging mental health survivors, consumers and service users through its radical politics of mental health, is now available online and uses a blog for communicating issues and events more widely.[5] With some online content explanatory for general viewers and readers, and other content speaking to communities of people affected by mental illness, the open and online world of interactions has power and possibility as a platform for action, as well as offering resources and support to those seeking help.

Mary O'Hagan told me that we had to ask, 'what's the story?' The overarching 'story' of madness and its multiple histories is one about those who were institutionalised, and what happened to them in the mental health system. My own response to this sense that we have failed to sufficiently engage the community of service users has been to start a project to engage with the field of mad histories. We need to engage with the personal stories and narratives of people who were institutionalised in psychiatric institutions in the twentieth century. Like O'Hagan, I agree that a 'much richer resource of material comes from a perspective of people who go through these experiences' (O'Hagan 2014, 24).

How do we do this work? One potential methodology is found in the idea of 'standing alongside' advocated by researchers interested in contemporary histories and communities including the histories of out of home care, adoption, child sexual abuse, and other histories.[6] By working with those who experienced history, we will gain an opportunity to critically analyse the way stories of mental illness are told, their relative power or meaning in our understandings of mental health treatment, and why they might help us to amplify many decades of histories of psychiatry and mental health.

This new conversation between medical personnel and psychiatrists and those with lived experience of mental illness will allow a more complete historical understanding. But this approach is not uncontroversial; to claim that we can collaborate across these spheres of medical models and experiences of madness highlights potential pitfalls. Negotiating the relationship between modalities of health and medicine, treatment and care, will be part of the future. That lies outside the scope of my own expertise, but my sense as a historian—as articulated here—is that talking, listening and hearing the points of view of the mad will go a long way towards shifting the conversation about what it means to experience mental illness.

What are the future directions for research and writing? The current energy around critical disability studies has fostered a new field of consumer, survivor-led writing and mad studies. For me, this must speak to the decades of historical work that has sought to enter into the worlds of the insane through available records; Reaume's inspirational study was part of a vanguard of social histories of madness that have shaped ways of thinking about future historical writing, setting us on the path of recognising the power relations of the institutions of the past. Realised in some of the events listed in Appendix A, this mission includes pulling apart the layers of madness as ahistorical and cultural, geographical experience. 'Madness: Probing the Boundaries' (Oxford, September 2014) was one symposium that offered different approaches to the topic including those presented by people with 'first-hand experience' of madness. Once, this inclusive style would have been unthinkable, even deemed impossible, by event organisers.

This event included seven themes for presenters, such as 'madness and the emotions'. The affective turn in history also holds much potential. How historians can evoke, communicate and represent the emotional worlds of the past is a challenge, and one that lends itself to psychology, health studies and creative collaborations. The 'Mad Love' asylum tapped into a rich vein of visualisation of spatial and physical experiences that shape our affective responses to states of mental wellbeing. We need to tell a new story of madness in public. Evidence suggests that reactions to personal stories of institutional confinement can transform our present understandings of mental health and mental illness; we know that storytelling has been acknowledged as playing an important part in social change. In the present, there is a social movement for the restoration of human rights to the institutionalised. Past injustices need to be addressed, not only in public forums, in documentaries, in published accounts of institutional life worlds, and in museum exhibitions, but also through action and advocacy.

Finally, histories that need to be researched and written with transnational teams of scholars include the story of aftercare across places, and the development of community psychiatry in a global perspective. Without hesitation, this field of historical studies continues as a truly international and interdisciplinary inquiry: the crisis in global mental health forces our sharp focus on what we might learn from the past, and especially from those people who have lived through their own periods of mental illness, and can reflect on that. Talking about madness, then, will always be vital to our recovery and resilience.

NOTES

1. https://wellcomecollection.org/pages/Wuw0uiIAACZd3SO0. Accessed 24 July 2019.
2. https://wellcomelibrary.org/collections/digital-collections/mental-healthcare/. Accessed 24 July 2019.
3. Victorian Parliamentary Papers (VPP), Kew Inquiry, *Minutes of Evidence*, Q 8120, Q 8122, p. 241.
4. https://news-archive.hud.ac.uk/news/2016/september/voicesofmadnessconferenceattractsaworldwideaudience.php. Accessed 14 July 2019.
5. See https://asylummagazine.org/. Accessed 16 July 2019.
6. See for example https://www.childabuseroyalcommission.gov.au/media-releases/research-reveals-dark-history-childrens-institutions-australia.

Suggested Readings

Clements, Judi. 2015. Lock-em up attitude is inappropriate. *Waikato Times.* April 29.

Coleborne, Catharine. 2018. Madness uncontained. In *Containing madness: Gender and 'psy' in institutional contexts*, eds Jennifer M. Kilty and Erin Dej, v–viii. Cham, Switzerland: Palgrave Macmillan.

Davies, Kerry. 2001. "Silent and censured travellers"? Patients' narratives and patients' voices: Perspectives on the history of mental illness since 1948. *Social History of Medicine* 14 (2): 267–292.

McCarthy et al. 2017. Lives in the asylum record, 1864 to 1910: Utilising large data collection for histories of psychiatry and mental health in the British World. *Medical History* 61 (3): 358–379.

O'Hagan, Mary. 2014. *Madness made me: A memoir.* Wellington: Open Box.

Porter, Roy. 2002. *Madness: A brief history.* Oxford: Oxford University Press.

Porter, Roy. 2004. The historiography of medicine in the United Kingdom. In *Locating medical history: The stories and their meanings*, eds Frank Huisman and John Harley Warner, 194–221. Baltimore: Johns Hopkins University Press.

Rothman, Sheila. 1994. *Living in the shadow of death: Tuberculosis and the social experience of illness in American history.* New York: Basic Books.

Tomes, Nancy. 1990. Historical perspectives on women and mental illness. In *Women, health and medicine in America: A historical handbook*, ed. Rima D. Apple, 143–171. New York and London: Garland Publishing.

Wong, Qiujing. 2015. How telling stories can bring social change. *New Zealand Herald*, April 27.

Documentaries and Digital Stories

Borderless Productions. 2014. Alison: 50 years under the system. http://borderless.co.nz/work/digital-storytelling/alisons-story/. Accessed March 2019.

Marbrook, Jim. 2012. Mental notes (Documentary). New Zealand. https://www.imdb.com/title/tt2076270/. Accessed 31 July 2019.

Appendix A: Mad Studies Conferences, Symposia and Events, 2014–2019

'Madness beyond psychiatry: A comparative and interdisciplinary study of mental disorder in Africa'. European Centre for African Studies. University of Edinburgh, UK. 10–14 June 2019.

'Around the humanities: Madness'. Centre for Interdisciplinary Studies in the Humanities and Social Sciences Student Council. Jagiellonian University, Poland. 27–28 April 2019.

'Developing mad studies'. Northeast Modern Language Association. New York, US. 21–24 March 2019.

'Mediating mental health: Lived experiences, mad studies and inter-disciplinary opportunities'. University of Canberra, Australia. 28 November 2018.

'Disability studies conference: "Mad Studies"'. Centre for Disability Research. Lancaster University, UK. 11–13 September 2018.

'Madness, mental illness and mind doctors in 20th and 21st century pop culture interdisciplinary conference'. University of Edinburgh, UK. 3–4 May 2018.

'From the margins to the center: Disability studies in other disciplines'. University of Chicago, US. 20–21 April 2018.

'Critical perspectives on and beyond activism and acts of resistance'. University College, Cork, Ireland. 9–10 November 2016.

C. Coleborne, *Why Talk About Madness?* Mental Health in Historical Perspective, https://doi.org/10.1007/978-3-030-21096-0

'Voices of Madness'. Centre for Health Histories. University of Huddersfield, UK. 15–16 July 2016.

'Disabilities studies conference: "Mad Studies"'. Centre for Disability Research. Lancaster University, UK. 6–8 September 2016.

'Making sense of madness'. Oxford University. UK. 10–12 July 2016.

'Driving us crazy'. International film festival organised in conjunction with Mad in America. Gothenburg, Sweden. 16–18 October 2015.

'Making sense of mad studies'. Centre for Medical Humanities. Durham University, UK. 30 September–1 October 2015.

'Colonising Madness: Postcolonial theory within critical disability studies, mad studies, and critical (educational) psychology'. University of Sheffield, UK. 14 September 2015.

'Disability, austerity and resistance'. University of NSW, Australia. 5 August 2015.

'Disability and disciplines: The international conference on educational, cultural and disability studies'. Liverpool Hope University, UK. 1–2 July 2015.

'Mad studies and neurodiversity: Exploring connections'. Lancaster University, UK. 17 June 2015.

'PsychoPolitics in the twenty first century: Peter Sedgwick and radical movements in mental health'. Liverpool Hope University, UK. 10 June 2015.

'Nordic network for disability research'. Bergen, Norway. May 2015.

'Making mad studies: Process, practice and contestations'. Ryerson University, Canada. 29 April 2015.

'Disabilities studies conference: "Mad Studies"'. Lancaster University, UK. 9–11 September 2014.

'Alternative psychiatric narratives'. Birkbeck. University of London, UK. 16–17 May 2014.

Appendix B: Mad Studies Networks and Social Media

Australia

International Disability Human Rights Network. https://research. unimelb.edu.au/hallmark-initiatives/home/disability/outcomes/ networks/disability-human-rights-research-network.

Off the Wall Inc. Critical Perspectives on 'Madness' Reading Group Humanist Society. http://www.offthewall.net.au/reading-groups/ https://www.meetup.com/en-AU/Critical-Perspectives-on-Madness-Reading-Group/.

Our Consumer Place: Resource centre for mental health consumers. http://www.ourconsumerplace.com.au/consumer/aboutus.

The MHS Learning Network NSW Australia. https://www.themhs.org/ about-themhs/.

Canada

Mad Students Society. http://madstudentsociety.com/.

The History of Madness in Canada. http://historyofmadness.ca/.

C. Coleborne, *Why Talk About Madness?* Mental Health in Historical Perspective, https://doi.org/10.1007/978-3-030-21096-0

Europe

Beautiful Distress Blog. https://www.beautifuldistress.org/blog/stigma-column-4-mad-studies-mek3k.

Stichting Perceval the Netherlands. http://www.madstudies.nl/.

United Kingdom

Asylum Blog: Asylum Magazine. http://asylummagazine.org/blog/.

Disabilities Studies Network: Mad Studies Reading Group, University of Edinburgh. https://www.disabilitystudiesnetwork.gla.ac.uk/2018/12/13/mad-studies-reading-group-edinburgh/.

Mad Studies North East. http://madstudiesne.weebly.com/.

North East Mad Studies Network and Forum. https://madstudies2014.wordpress.com/.

Pink Sky Thinking Mad Studies Group (LXP Focus), University of Birmingham. https://www.pinkskythinking.com/post/introducing-a-mad-studies-group-in-birmingham.

Powys Mental Health Blog, PAVO Wales. http://powysmentalhealth.blogspot.com/2015/12/making-sense-of-mad-studies.html.

United States

Mad in America. https://www.madinamerica.com/2018/06/introducing-new-mad-studies-webinar-series/.

NeuroDIVERSITY and Inclusion: Mad Studies Podcast. https://sites.duke.edu/neurodiversityandinclusion/videos/mad-studies-podcast/.

Facebook, You Tube, Twitter

Mad Studies Network. https://www.facebook.com/groups/394088527441084/.

Beresford, Peter. 2 July 2015. From Psychiatry to Disability Studies and Mad Studies. https://www.youtube.com/watch?v=romAt_o3-Vo.

Ingram, Richard. 13 June 2016. Making Sense of Mad Studies Parts 1 and 2. https://www.youtube.com/watch?v=HrPyE1b-cEk https://www.youtube.com/watch?v=RNBF8UiH17I.

Mad Studies Birmingham Pilot Meeting. 8 February 2019. https://www.youtube.com/watch?v=Kj5dco4RUkw.

Mad Studies. 21 June 2016. https://www.youtube.com/watch?v=6Vsw
    4WjuUTE.
@Mad_In_America.   January   2012.   https://twitter.com/mad_in_
    america?lang=en.
#madisnotbad. https://twitter.com/hashtag/madisnotbad?src=hash.
#MadPride. https://twitter.com/hashtag/MadPride?src=hash.
#MadStudies. https://twitter.com/hashtag/madstudies?src=hash.

INDEX

A

Aboriginal, 2, 21, 60

Aboriginal child removal, 60

Abuse, 17, 51, 59–60, 63, 70

Adam Art Gallery (Wellington, New Zealand), 33, 35, 37

advocacy, v, ix, 3, 5, 10, 24, 34, 45, 47–8, 53–9, 71

Africa, 18, 22, 73

aftercare, 44–5, 50, 55, 71. *See also* extra-institutional care

Aftercare Association (New South Wales, Australia), 45

Aftercare Association of Poor and Friendless Female Convalescents (England), 45

Allen, Hannah, 7

anti-psychiatry, 2, 4, 9, 42, 45–7

architecture, 35

asylum archive, 15–28

asylum
  furniture, 32
  records of, 4–9, 15–26
  routines, 17, 30, 59
  spaces, 25, 29, 30, 32–37
  staff, 15, 30, 58

Asylum Magazine, 51n, 69, 76

Australia, 1, 3, 8, 11, 18, 20–1, 30, 43, 45, 47–8, 55, 60, 67, 68

autobiography, 7–8

B

Basaglia, Franco, 46

Bedlam, 15, 30, 32

Benjamin, Jonny, 61

Britain, 1, 22, 48, 49, 56

British Columbia (Canada), 21

British world, 1, 3, 18

Browne, W. A. F., 36

Brownless Medical Museum (Melbourne), 34

C

Canada, 1, 3, 18, 20, 46, 48, 55, 61, 68

Caribbean, 18

Charles Brothers Collection, 34, 37n

China, 43

© The Editor(s) (if applicable) and The Author(s), under exclusive license to Springer Nature Switzerland AG 2020

C. Coleborne, *Why Talk About Madness?* Mental Health in Historical Perspective, https://doi.org/10.1007/978-3-030-21096-0

Clark, Helen, 58
Class, 9, 18, 20, 23–4, 43
closure, ix, 1, 3, 5, 9, 30–3, 35, 37,
    41, 50, 54, 57–8, 61, 65. *See also*
    deinstitutionalisation
Colney Hatch, 6. *See also* Friern
colonisation, 3, 69
Commission to Inquire into Child
    Abuse (Ireland, 2000–2009), 60
Commonwealth, 3
community care, 33, 44–9, 56–7
Confidential Forum for Former
    In-Patients of Psychiatric
    Hospitals in New Zealand
    (2004–2006), 53–61
Crichton Royal Institution (Dumfries,
    Scotland), 36–7

D
Dax, Eric Cunningham, 47
deinstitutionalisation, 1, 31–3, 41, 48,
    54, 56–7. *See also* closure
diagnoses, 1, 8, 16, 18
digital communication, 16, 68
disability, 59, 68, 70
documentary, 10, 56, 67

E
ethnicity, 18, 20, 23–4
extra-institutional care, 9, 41–51. *See
    also* aftercare

F
families, 9, 11, 22–3, 24, 41, 42–4,
    58, 65
Fanon, Frantz, 46
Fiji, 18
filmmakers, 10. *See also* documentary
Foucault, Michel, 3, 4, 16, 46

Frame, Janet, 8
France, 43
Freud, Sigmund, 7
Friern, 6. *See also* Colney Hatch

G
gender, 9, 11, 18, 20, 29. *See also*
    transgender
Gheel, Belgium, 42–3
Gilman, Charlotte Perkins, 8
Gilman, Sander, 16
Gittins, Diana, 3–4
global mental health, 2, 11, 71
Goffman, Erving, 29–30, 46
Gould Farm (Berkshires), 43
graffiti, 32

H
Hanwell Asylum (Middlesex), 15
Hartwood Hospital (Scotland), 47
'Hearing Voices', 2
Helm, Anne, 59
heredity, 20
heritage, 30
Holocaust, 5

I
Imperial War Museum, 30
India, 18
Industrialisation, 18, 20
intellectual disability, 59
Ireland, 43, 55, 68
Italy, 43

J
Japan, 43
Jones, Kathleen, 46

K
Kew Metropolitan Asylum (Victoria, Australia), 30
Kingsley Hall (London), 46

L
labour, 18, 20
legislation, 54–55
leisure, 9, 17
lived experience, 32, 33, 36, 47, 49, 67–70

M
'Mad Love', 32, 71
Mad Pride, 48
mad studies, 2, 53, 68, 73–6
Mason Report (New Zealand), 57
material culture, 10, 19, 20, 32–3, 36, 68
mental health advocates, 1, 59
Mental Health and Wellbeing Commission (New Zealand), 61
Mental Health Association (Australia), 47
Mental Health Commissioner (New Zealand), 6
Mental Health Foundation
  of Australia, 47; of New Zealand, 60
mental health movement, 4, 47
Mental Health Rights Coalition (Ontario, Canada), 48
mental health service user, 4, 9, 10, 24
Mental Hygiene Authority (Victoria, Australia), 47
Mental Patients' Association (Vancouver, Canada), 48
#MeToo, 5
Museum of Brisbane, 35
Museums Victoria, 34

N
New York State Museum, 35
New Zealand, 1, 3, 6, 18, 20–3, 32–3, 35, 43–8, 53–63, 67–8
Norway, 43

O
O'Hagan, Mary, 6, 16, 48, 56, 66, 69
open care, 42–3, 46
oral narrative, 7, 58
outsider art, 36

P
Packard, Elizabeth, 8
pathography, 10, 22
peer support, 45, 48–9, 67
photography, 10, 22
Plath, Sylvia, 8
Porirua Hospital (New Zealand), 58
Porter, Roy, 1, 2, 19, 45–6, 68
poverty, 17, 18, 20, 23–4, 49
psychiatric survivor, 2, 4–5, 9, 22, 37, 46–8, 56, 61, 67–8, 70
psychoanalysts, 46
psychology, 70

R
Reaume, Geoffrey, 10, 17, 19, 56, 70
restraints, 18, 34, 37
Rose, Diana, 48

S
Sacks, Oliver, 4, 32
schizophrenia, 46
Scottish Union of Mental Patients, 47
Scull, Andrew, 2, 13n, 21, 29, 30
Severalls Hospital, 3
social psychiatry, 46

sources, 19, 22, 25, 32, 34
  case notes, 4, 16, 24
  diaries, 66
  letters, 7, 19, 22, 65, 66, 67
  patient records, 22
South Africa, 18, 22
Spandler, Helen, 47, 49
stigma, 6, 9, 23, 54, 57, 59–60, 61
storytelling, 10, 25, 67–71
suicide, 7, 11
Suzuki, Akihito, 42–3
Szasz, Thomas, 4

T
Taylor, Barbara, 6, 33, 45
Te Awamutu Museum (New Zealand),
  35–6
therapeutic community, 46
Tokanui Hospital, 3, 23, 35, 46, 57–8
Tomes, Nancy, 42
'total institution', 5, 29, 30
transgender, 59
treatments

electro-convulsive therapy (ECT),
  24, 58
solitary confinement, 23

U
United Nations, 6
United States, 43, 55, 68

W
welfare, 20, 47, 49, 60
Wellcome Collection, 40n
  exhibition, 32, 71
Wellcome Library, 15
Wellcome Trust, 48, 65
Weyburn Mental Hospital (Canada),
  46
Whai Ora, 3
Wood, Mary Elene, 7
World Health Organization, 2, 6
World Network of Users and Survivors
  of Psychiatry, 6

CPSIA information can be obtained
at www.ICGtesting.com
Printed in the USA
LVHW080751020720
659485LV00014B/348